ENDOMETRIOSIS
NATURALLY
COOKBOOK

with 131 Recipes

ENDOMETRIOSIS NATURALLY COOKBOOK

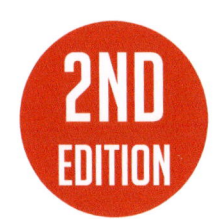
2ND EDITION

with **131** Recipes

WENDY K LAIDLAW

©Copyright 2022 Wendy K Laidlaw

All Rights Reserved.

ISBN-13: 979 883 277 2769

No part of this publication may be reproduced, distributed, or transmitted in any form or by any means, including photocopying, recording or other electronic or mechanical methods, without the express prior written permission of the author, except in the case of brief quotations embodied in critical reviews and certain other noncommercial uses permitted by copyright law.

For all permissions and requests please write to the **EndoBoss®Team** at Support@HealEndometriosisNaturally.zohodesk.com

Visit www.HealEndometriosisNaturally.com for more specialist support and information.

Recipes curated by Wendy K Laidlaw and Sebastian C N Anderson

Edited by Maxine I K Anderson and Sebastian C N Anderson

Cover design by Salman Sarwar, Sam Art Studio
Interior design by Liliana Gonzalez Garcia

Wendy's photograph by Nate Cleary

Other Books by Wendy K Laidlaw   Heal Endometriosis Naturally

- How I Ended My Endometriosis Naturally; Without Painkillers, Drugs or Surgery (2021)
- Morning Wisdom Journal Writing Your Way To Health (2021)

TESTIMONIALS

This Cookbook is a treasure trove!

"Wow! I had no idea this cookbook was so thorough. It covers so many excellent recipes. I have zero complaints. Tonight I'm cooking up the salmon dish! I can't wait to try it. Wendy has done an amazing job organizing the perfect recipes for women struggling with endometriosis. I could not be more grateful for the immense amount of time she must have put into developing this book. What a blessing it is for all of us. I also LOVE the fact that she lays out her own story and philosophy behind these foods in the beginning of her book. It really helps me to understand why she recommends these foods and why it's so important we stick to the plan! Thank you Wendy! Bravo!"

Kris L, Amazon Review

When you are tired of being tired

"WOW! Thank you. This cook book is for those who are tired of being tired. Food that heals. Recipes are easy to make and delicious. Great photos. A must purchase for those who want to support the healing of their bodies with food first and not drugs."

Amazon Customer Review

Healthy eating made easy!

"I don't have endometriosis, but this is a great book even if you just want to eliminate toxins from your diet. I don't like cooking/spending a lot of time on food prep, so this provides practical, efficient and easy to follow recipes! I'm inspired to be healthy, while still enjoying delicious food-especially the healthy options for muffins and sweet treats! There's also a super helpful shopping list at the start of the book-you then have all of the ingredients ready to go, rather than having to buy special ingredients for 'one off recipes'. The inspirational quotes are also a nice touch throughout, they remind you of the benefits of healthy eating and help keep you on track! Thanks to the author, this is a great collection of recipes!"

Rachel McKinnon, Amazon Review

Fantastic book-couldn't be better!

"The recipes are easy and very tasty-the best thing about them is that all my family thought the same and didn't notice that there was anything different to what we normally eat. To cure yourself you need to buy her other book too-she does know what she's talking about unlike most people. Buy them both and transform your life!"

Amazon Customer Review

MEDICAL DISCLAIMER

This book should not be used in place of professional medical advice and nor should the information be treated as professional medical advice.

This book is based on Wendy's personal experiences and what worked for her on her healing journey. What she shares are the principles that have helped her on her journey, alongside specific recipes to help guide you further.

These principles have been derived from over 30 years worth of her own healing journey experiences and processes that led to her full recovery from the pain and symptoms of endometriosis (and adenomyosis). She has also read and studied a great deal on the subject of endometriosis, and been qualified in the field of nutritional therapy. However, she is making no claims and cannot promise that this book will work for every woman.

If you have any specific questions about any medical matter you should consult your doctor or other professional healthcare provider.

The author advises readers to take full responsibility for all of their decisions, particularly with regards to their body and health.

If you think you may be suffering from any medical condition, worsening of symptoms or any new symptoms that are not resolving, you should seek immediate medical attention and insist symptoms are investigated by tests that are beyond the scope of this book.

You should never delay seeking medical advice, disregard medical advice, or discontinue medical treatment because of the information presented in this or any other book.

Please use this book responsibly. The author does not take any responsibility for anybody who misuses the advice suggested in here.

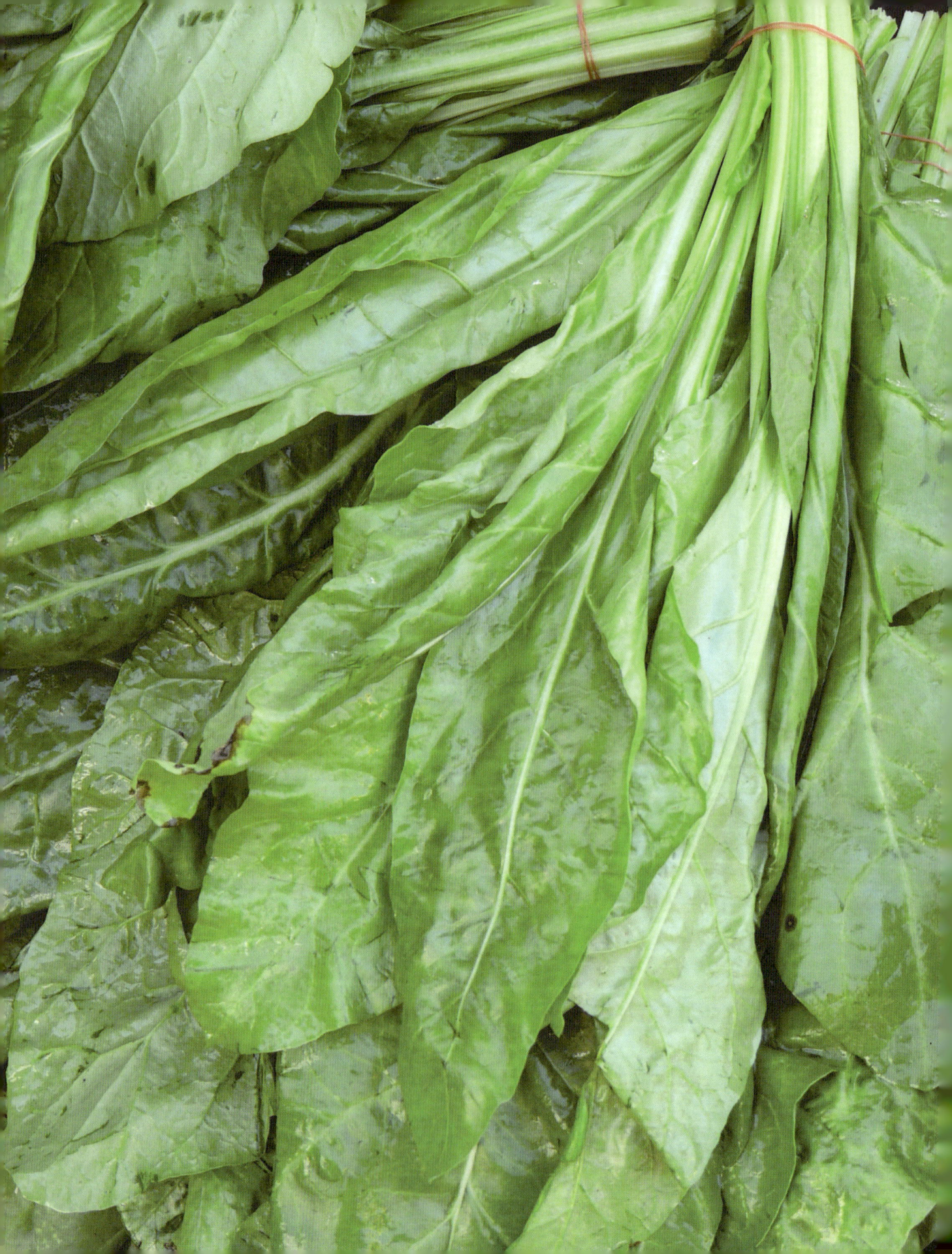

DEDICATIONS

I dedicate this fully updated and revised 2nd edition cookbook to my darling adult children; Maxine & Sebastian.

Gynecologists repeatedly told me over many years that I would never have any children, so I am so grateful at having them in my life and the fine people they have become.

Both Maxine and Sebastian regularly and generously commit countless hours of their free time to assist me in my mission to inspire and educate women globally about how women can become an EndoBoss®. I love that helping women with endometriosis to heal naturally is now our family mission.

Maxine and Sebastian; **thank you** for all that you do to assist me in spreading this important message of hope and healing.

Keep journaling, eating healthily, chewing thoroughly and let food be your medicine!

I love you both so much with all of my heart and soul.

All my love always,

Mum xx

Secondly, I dedicate this cookbook to all the future EndoBosses. You have everything inside of you to take back power and control of this condition and become a boss of endometriosis; an **EndoBoss®**!

I look forward to hearing about your successful journey soon.

Wendy xx

"The natural healing force within each one of us is the greatest force in getting well.

Our food should be our medicine. Our medicine should be our food."

— HIPPOCRATES

ENDOBOSS® STUDENTS & ALUMNI **SPECIAL MENTIONS**

Well done to some of our wonderful EndoBosses who have contributed some of their favorite recipes to this 2nd edition cookbook.

Congratulations to Jessica Le Gray, Rachel Sledge, Marie West, Anita Clohesy, Natalie Krier, Nadja Ilic and Laura Majugo for winning a place for their recipes within this updated book.

These incredible women were successful participants of my Heal Endometriosis Naturally, **EndoBoss® Academy Program** and other Programs and have made the necessary commitment and changes to become a boss of their endometriosis; an EndoBoss®!

I am so super proud of you all so make sure to keep working the 3 Daily Basics and, of course, keep paying close attention to the Five Poisons (5 Ps) to keep your condition in remission.

Keep up the excellent work on yourself.

You are all incredible women.

To your health,

Wendy xx

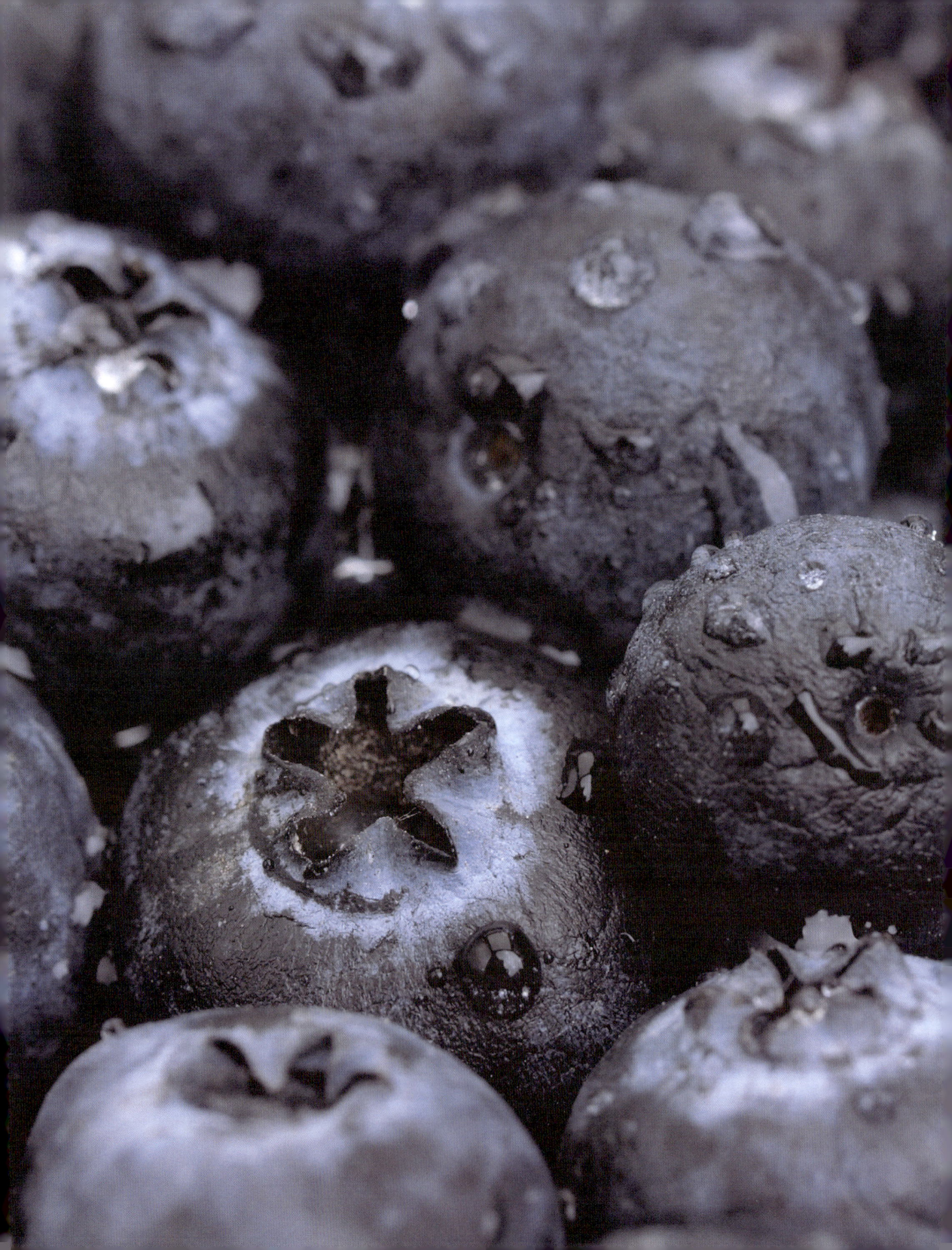

ACKNOWLEDGEMENTS

I would like to say a *huge* thank you to my wonderful business coach and dear friend, Christian Fioravanti, for his unwavering kindness, generosity of spirit, guidance and support over the past few years.

Christian has been instrumental in guiding me through the internet maze. He has enabled me to safely share my journey, healing story and message of hope to the millions of women around the world who are suffering needlessly with endometriosis.

Already my other books and online programs are helping to transform tens of thousands of womens lives for the better and helps them tap into their unique infinite power and strength to heal their endometriosis naturally.

Christian thank you. You have been such an incredible star and gift to the world.

Thank you for all the good work you do in the world as well. I could not have got this far without you.

Warmest regards,

Wendy xx

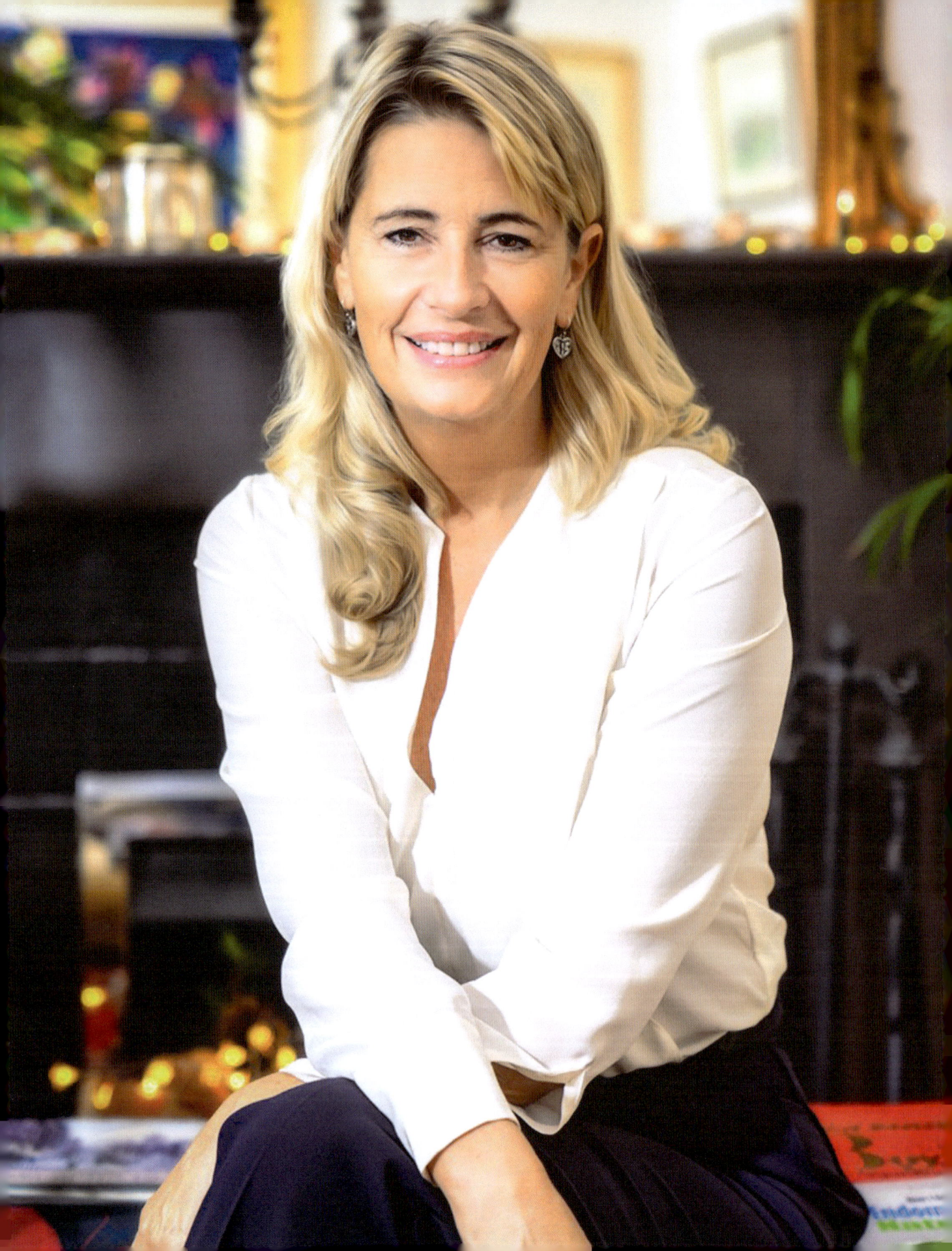

MEET WENDY K LAIDLAW

I am a women's health pioneer and the world's leading expert on healing endometriosis naturally. I am the founder and CEO of HealEndometriosisNaturally, an international multi-best selling author, an online summit host and the creator of the No.1 endometriosis podcast: 'Heal Endometriosis Naturally With Wendy K Laidlaw'.

I have been featured on over 36 national radio stations including the BBC, and appeared in publications such as Authority Magazine and Vogue Magazine and I have also been featured on the cover of Brainz Magazine.

As a visionary and thought leader in women's pelvic health, my mission is to revolutionise and modernise the gynaecological field worldwide.

But, what makes me 'qualified' to help women with endometriosis?

Well, I suffered from stage IV endometriosis for **over 33 years**. It dominated and controlled my world to the point that I had no life. For three decades I tried the usual ways of healing that were touted by doctors and consultants. I had six surgeries, countless drugs and thousands of painkillers but only continued to get worse.

My pain became unbearable and my symptoms even more complex. My insides were wracked with endless adhesions and multiple large chocolate cysts. I also developed a plethora of other conditions including fibromyalgia, glandular fever, adenomyosis, and chronic fatigue syndrome.

The conventional medical system failed me and I ended up bedridden for almost three years.

During this dark and dire time, something within me refused to give up, and following some enlightening encounters and realisations, I became convinced that there had to be a way out of this illness, misery and pain. I thought that the body is always wanting to heal, so what was preventing mine?

Bedridden for over 2 years and cradling my hot water bottle, fighting through the pain, I researched desperately from my bed and began a journey of learning and self-discovery. I trained in nutritional therapy, psychotherapy and psychology, and became a certified coach. I was on a mission to heal my body.

Over many months, I gradually pieced the elements that were responsible for my ill health. From this I developed a set of multi-model, holistic, science-based protocols, now called the Laidlaw Protocols. These helped to address the poisons (the 5 Ps) that were previously prohibiting my body's natural ability to heal. Following this pathway enabled me, after 10-12 months, to put all of my medical conditions into remission; naturally. To this day, over **6 years on**, I remain free from all the conditions, symptoms and pain I once had.

I have now dedicated the rest of my life to share with women all around the world, that endometriosis is not a life-sentence. My mission is to continue to empower women to recognise the power they have over their own bodies with the right information, education and inspiration.

This passion to educate women with endometriosis, and their emotions has led me to pioneer several impactful online programs and start to teach healthcare professionals in the effective and compassionate approaches required for true healing.

So why this book?

Well, the first element of the 5 Ps is Produce (what food we eat and drink).

So this cookbook is here to guide you on the first stage of sharing how to eat healthily and simply, whilst learning to listen to your body.

It is important to mention that the healing process requires a multi-model approach addressing all of the 5 Ps and not just Produce. So remember this new journey is not a quick fix.

However, I do expect that you will experience some alleviations or positive benefits from following the recipes and suggestions but allow at least 10-12 weeks.

This is because everything you eat directly affects your cells.

Any toxins or poisons you have consumed have to be dealt with and take time to be processed out of the body. Allow your amazing immune system to do what it is excellent at doing; which is to heal the body.

Our hunter-gathering cave women ancestors would have not grazed on poisonous processed foods, soy, seed oils and grains.

Whilst the human body is excellent at adaptation over the centuries, unfortunately toxins and poisons build up in the body and it struggles to process them.

So start slowly (slow is fast!) and be realistic about time frames and ability to swap out your current foods and habits. It's a marathon not a sprint!

Be kind and compassionate with yourself if you are just starting out and try to encourage your partner or family or a friend to join you for a few months. You will all notice the difference in monthly cycles, moods and energy levels.

Your aim is to eat as fresh and as close to nature as possible, meaning pasture-raised, hormone-free, grass-fed, organic foods wherever you can. It's nearly impossible to do it 100% but start off with realistic goals and congratulate yourself each time you increase your awareness of what you are eating and how your body is responding.

Let food be your medicine and feel the difference in your body!

Your health depends upon it.

Wendy xx

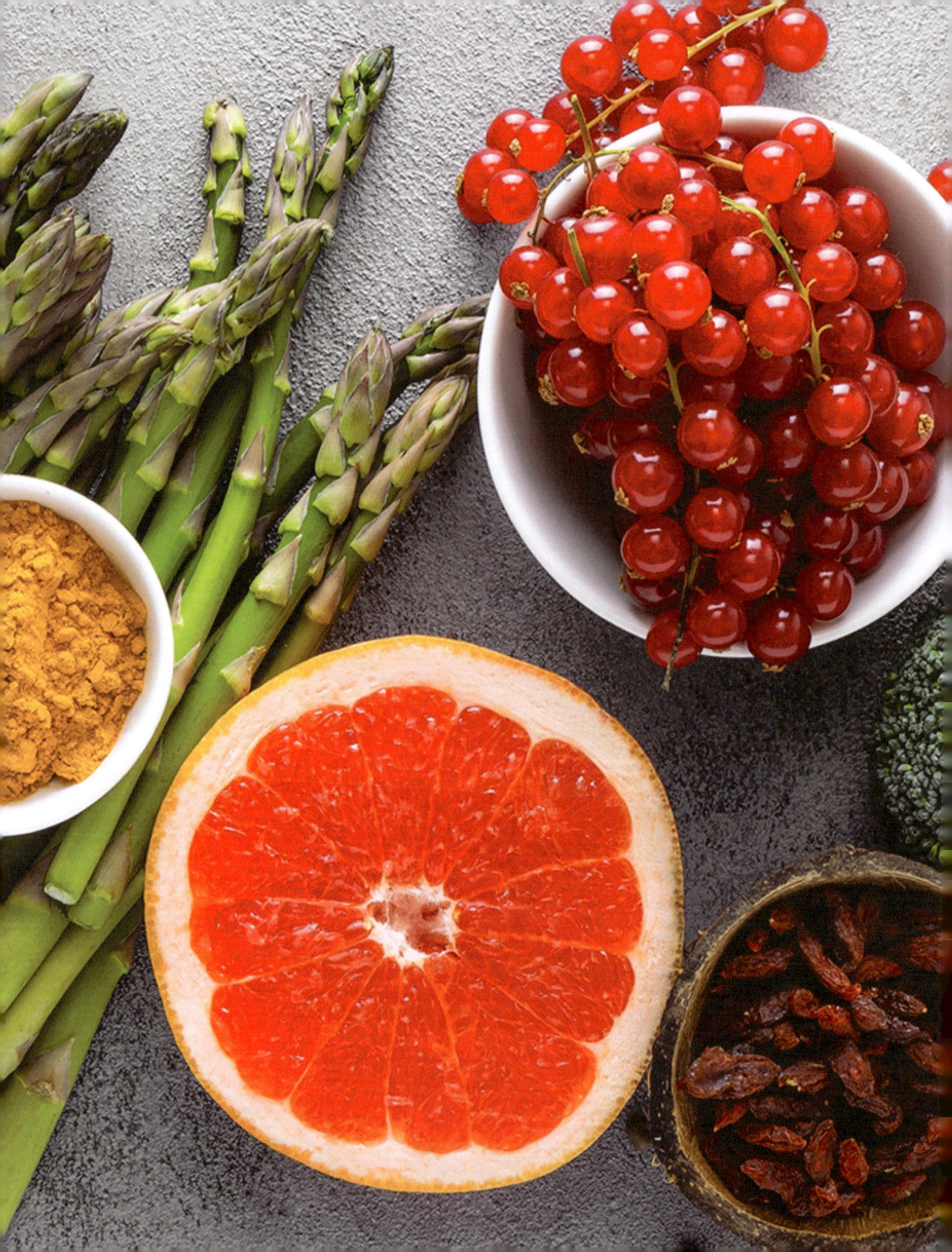

CONTENTS

MEET WENDY K LAIDLAW — **15**

MY FOOD PHILOSOPHY — **21**

THE GOOD FOOD GUIDELINES — **23**

FOOD COMBINING: EATING THE RIGHT FOODS IN ORDER — **29**

REMOVE & REPLACE FOR THE NEXT 12 WEEKS — **31**

HOW FOOD IS 'MADE' IN OUR MODERN WORLD — **35**

SHOPPING LIST — **37**

BREAKFAST LIKE A QUEEN — **41**

SMOOTHIES & JUICES — **69**

LUSCIOUS LUNCHES & SALADS — **99**

DELICIOUS DINNERS & MAINS — **123**

SUPER SCRUMPTIOUS SOUPS — **189**

PERFECTLY HEALTHY PUDDINGS — **219**

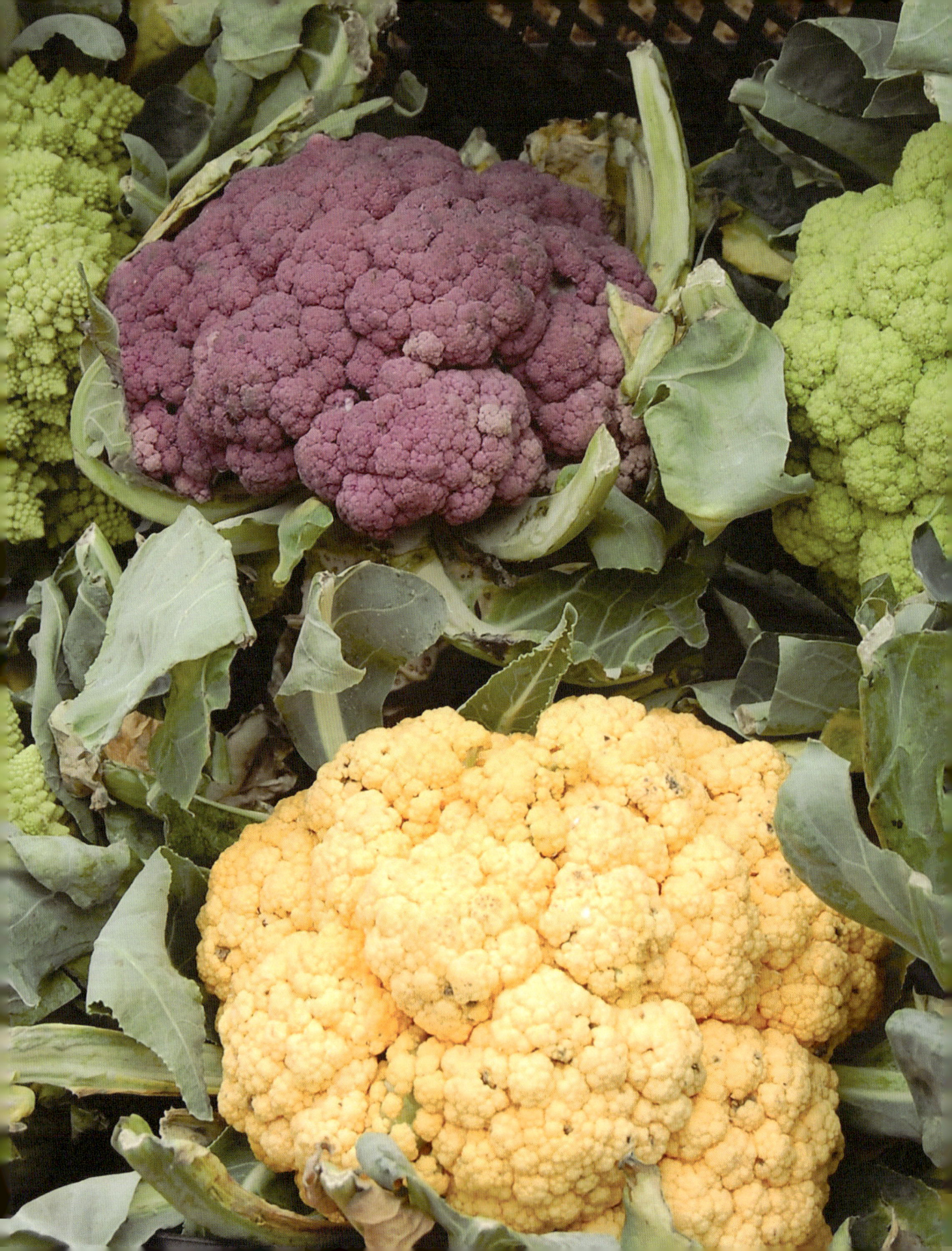

MY FOOD PHILOSOPHY

The KISS Principle-"Keeping It Super Simple"

My 'food philosophy' consists of a few simple guidelines. Follow them and within a few months, sometimes weeks, you may start to notice some positive differences in your body. Over many more months, and perhaps years, you will see even greater and more dramatic positive changes. Your body is an amazing self-healing organism given the right ingredients and environments.

When considering your purchases or meals ask yourself questions such as;

"Is this food something my Great Great Grandmother would have recognized as food?" or *"Would my hunter-gatherer ancestors have eaten this?."* Maybe question *"Could I or a local farmer have made/grown/ cultivated/farmed this food?"* or *"How many factory hands has this food been processed through before reaching me?"*

The aim is to keep increasing your awareness about what you eat and how your body feels afterwards. You are wanting to avoid the heavily processed food that is full of toxic or unnatural ingredients that are not found in nature or only accessible via intensive factory processing.

I am not a fan of 'diets' so we are swapping this word for **'Good Food Habits'** instead. The notion of a diet is emotive and insinuates that this eating pattern will be temporary or a short term fad. To get lasting results and full health, your eating needs to be a plan for life and it must become a part of your new EndoBoss® lifestyle.

Remember that new habits take time to develop and old ones take time to break. So, start super slowly by changing your foods a few at a time or addressing one meal a day and then build up from there.

If you change everything at once, your new eating habits may feel overwhelming, overly restrictive or like a punishment and this will most likely make them unsustainable. Also be mindful of your environments and toxic people in them which may trigger you into old patterns of eating (like craving artificial sugar after being around certain people).

Please do not get fixated on the number of calories or weighing food (hence why I talk in loose terms with quantities in recipes). Whilst they can be useful tools for other goals they are not necessary for your overall health here. You will be surprised at how much healthier and stronger your body becomes by getting focused on eating more simple, natural, unprocessed and fresh food.

Your taste buds, and body, will love it.

THE GOOD FOOD GUIDELINES

Guideline 1.

Eat As Much As You Like Of The Simple Foods

Use the 'KISS' Principle (Keeping It Super Simple) means eating foods that occur naturally in nature or that are as close to their original form as possible.

These foods will not be genetically modified (GMO) and are free from pesticides, chemicals, hormones, and sprays. If possible, these foods are seasonal and local. When it comes to identifying these foods, they may often be labelled as organic, grass-fed (red meat), pasture raised (chicken, eggs, pork), or fresh-caught (seafood).

Guideline 2.

Dump The Junk

Junk food is often very high in artificial sugar which releases endorphins and dopamine when consumed. This is why such foods can make you feel great immediately upon eating and then feel yuk and have a slump afterwards. However, too much sugar, especially when consumed without proper nutrients, may cause an increase in inflammation which may worsen the symptoms of endometriosis.

Almost all junk food, and even other more minimally processed foods, contain seed oils such as sunflower or rapeseed oil. These polyunsaturated fats are incredibly toxic to the body as they are very unstable and once in the body, can create a huge amount of inflammation. Junk food also contains a variety of other toxic components such as trans fats, colorants and preservatives.

Guideline 3.

Never Go Hungry!

Eat little and often as this helps to keep your blood sugar levels balanced and energy levels high throughout the day. It also ensures that your body is getting a steady supply of important nutrients such as protein.

Remember to plan and prepare your food consumption in advance for the next day; as my Grandmother used to say "If you fail to plan, you plan to fail."

Guideline 4.

Sit Down To Eat

Eating on the go or standing up to eat makes you more likely to rush consumption of your food and not chew it thoroughly, which may result in heartburn, indigestion, and/or bloating. By sitting down and taking time for your meals, you will be more focused on and appreciative of the food you are eating. Switch off your mobile phone and allow yourself at least 30 minutes of space which may make you feel more satiated and help with absorption and digestion.

Guideline 5.

Chew, Chew & CHEW Your Food (At Least 15-20 Times Each Mouthful)

Remember that your stomach has no teeth! Ensure you are chewing your food so it is almost a liquid, before swallowing. The primary function of your teeth is chewing to break down food so that your gastric juices can further break it down into smaller digestible molecules. Chewing also stimulates areas of the digestive system processes and helps expose your food to saliva. Swallowing any un-chewed food may lead to flatulence, bloating, belching and/or indigestion pain.

Guideline 6.

Variety Is The Spice Of Life

Get creative and have fun with your food, as eating well or healthily does not mean your food has to be dull or boring! Experiment with the ingredients and combinations suggested here and get in touch with your creativity. If you don't feel like eating at some parts of the day then consider 'drinking your food' instead with shakes, juices and soups.

Guideline 7.

If You Fail to Plan, You Plan to Fail

If your days are very busy or you are feeling ill or in chronic pain, then the idea of shopping, preparing, and cooking food may feel overwhelming. The main way around this is by planning ahead. This could mean scheduling an online food delivery once a week where you get healthy foods that can be used in simple, quick, and nutritious recipes like soups or one-pot dishes. Equally, planning may involve ordering healthy pre-prepared meals or food boxes. Planning can also include creating lists of easy, nutritious snacks and quick bites to eat so that when you are hungry, you don't have to stress or opt for something less nutritious. Also consider asking a safe friend to assist you with food when unwell.

Guideline 8.

Food, Feelings & Emotions

Your health and emotions are intricately linked to what you eat (for example, think why you are drawn to certain foods at certain times of stress; for many this is artificial sugar or chocolate). Become aware of how you feel physically and emotionally before and after eating certain food types. See if you are able to identify any patterns between certain foods, mealtimes, or situations. I suggest keeping a food journal at the back of your main Morning Pages journal to monitor this for a few weeks.

Guideline 9.

You Are What You Digest

What you eat is important but what you digest is paramount to absorbing essential nutrients. A significant portion of the world's population, particularly those under high levels of prolonged and unremitting stress, may not have enough stomach acid to break down food and destroy any pathogens or bacteria that come in through the mouth. This condition is known as hypochlorhydria. Having low or no stomach acid may cause issues in the full digestion of your food and thus inhibit the ability to extract important vitamins, minerals and amino acids from it. To test for this deficiency, I recommend a simple home test called The Baking Soda digestion test (see HealEndometriosisNaturally.com for details). If the results suggest that you have hypochlorhydria then consider slowly introducing a supplement called Betaine HCL with each meal. Taking digestive enzymes may also be a good addition to further assist you in breaking down your food effectively as your body heals. Live or raw food has its own digestive enzymes but processed or cooked food may require supplementation with digestive enzymes if you have poor digestion.

Guideline 10.

Give It 10-12 Months Minimum To See Lasting Improvements

Your amazing body will take time to heal so you must be patient when changing your daily eating habits. I suggest changing things over slowly so the changes will be gradual and take a few months to be felt and seen. If you follow the above recommendations (and additions in my 'How I Ended My Endometriosis Naturally' book) then you will see the benefits.

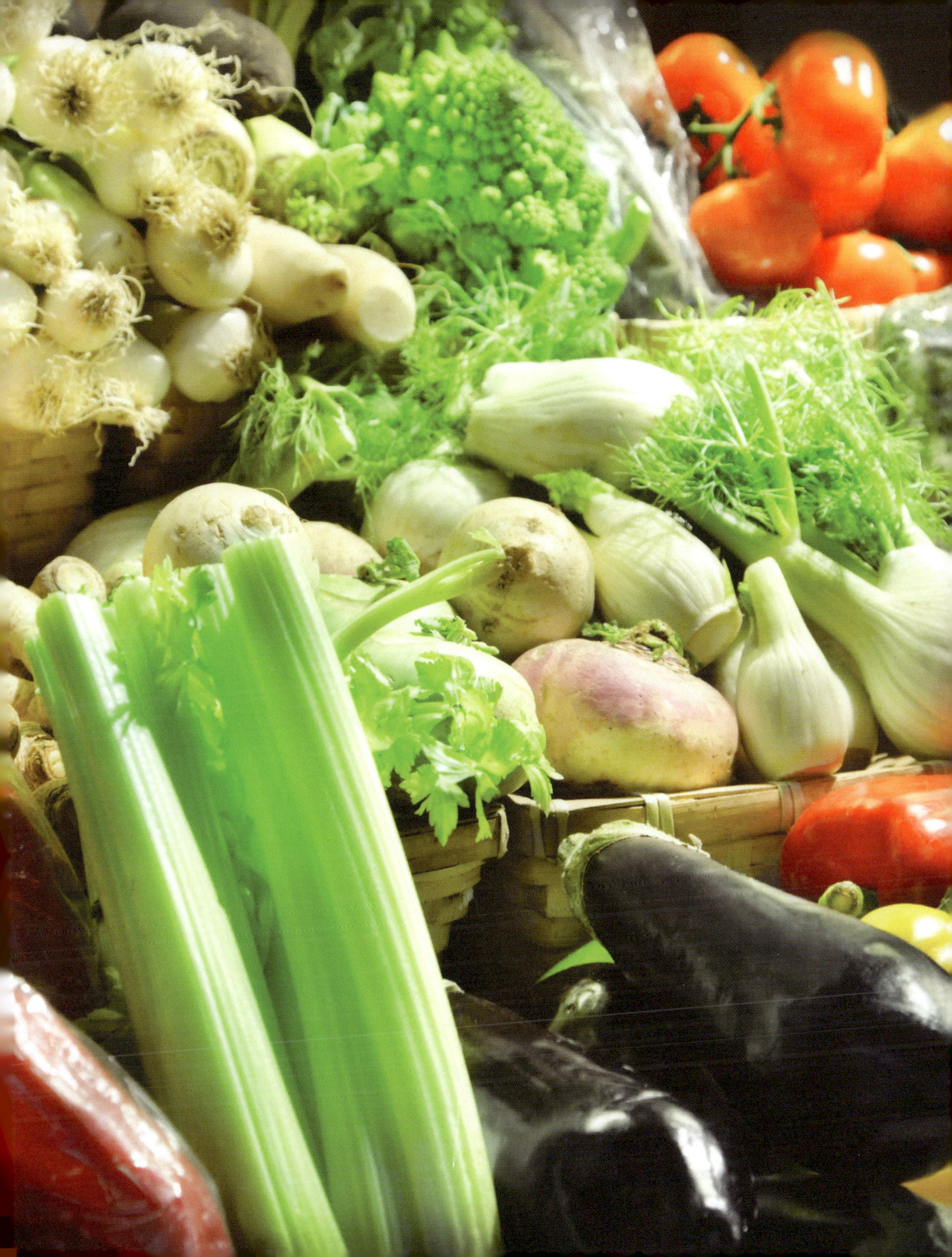

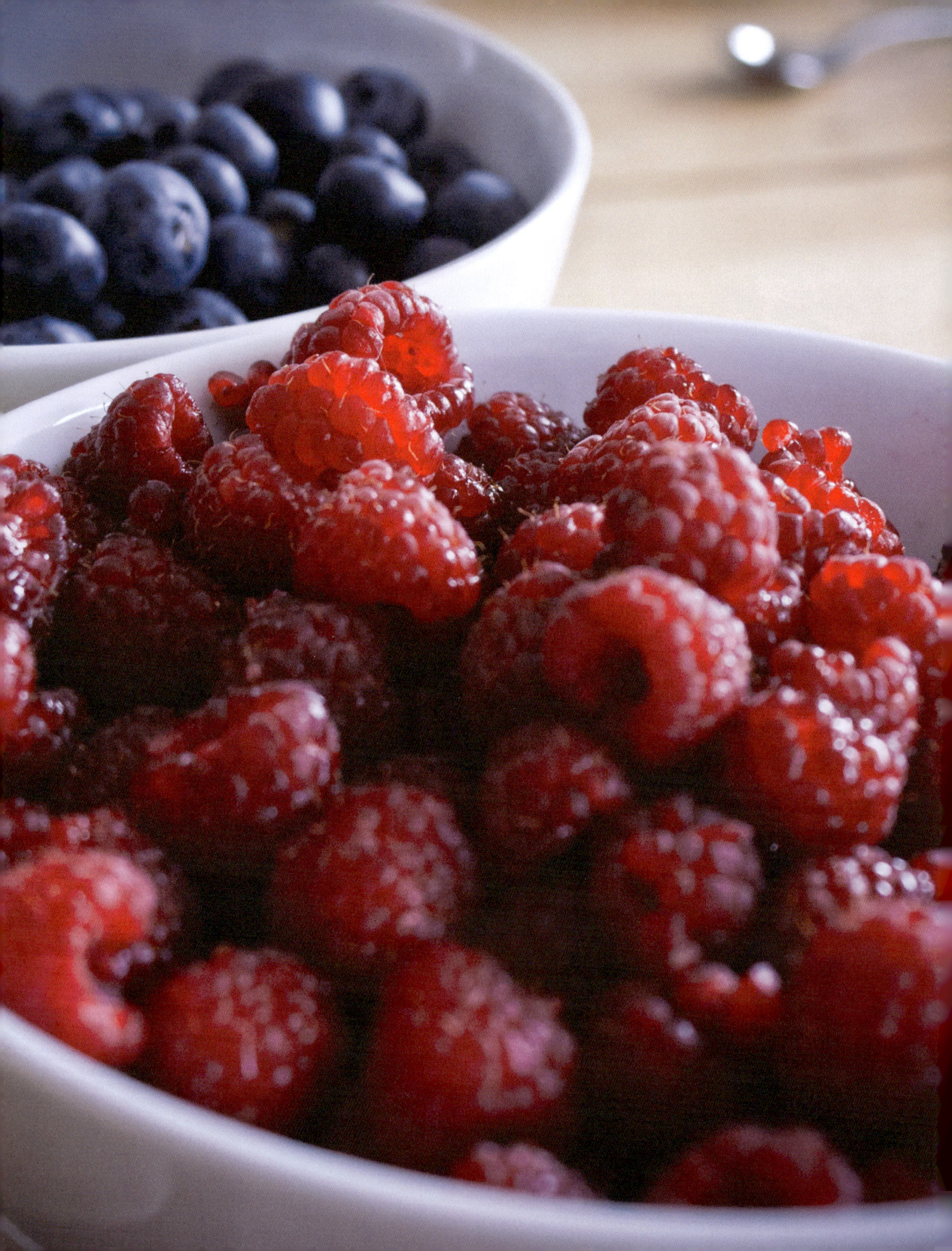

'FOOD COMBINING' EATING THE RIGHT FOODS IN ORDER

If you have tested your stomach acid levels and are supplementing with digestive enzymes but you are still experiencing discomfort, indigestion, gas and bloating, you may wish to consider the 'food combining' or 'food separating' approach to eating.

For example, make sure that you separate out the food groups during your meals (see the suggested guideline below).

Digestive Processing Time

Fruit	quickest	30 minutes
Carbohydrates	medium	60 minutes
Protein	longest	90 minutes

Consider eating fruit at least 30 minutes prior to eating any other food types if you feel your stomach and abdomen is very sensitive at times.

Then leave at least two hours AFTER eating a carbohydrate-based meal before eating any dense or solid protein meal like chicken, fish or meat.

Then leave three hours AFTER eating any solid protein source before eating carbohydrates.

Depending on where you are on your EndoBoss® journey remember that beans and pulses are combination of protein and starch, so are easily combined into salads. However, they may be troublesome for some women with endometriosis, so ensure to document and tune in to how your body responds after eating them and any other foods. Consider keeping a separate Food Journal to increase your awareness and new relationship with your body.

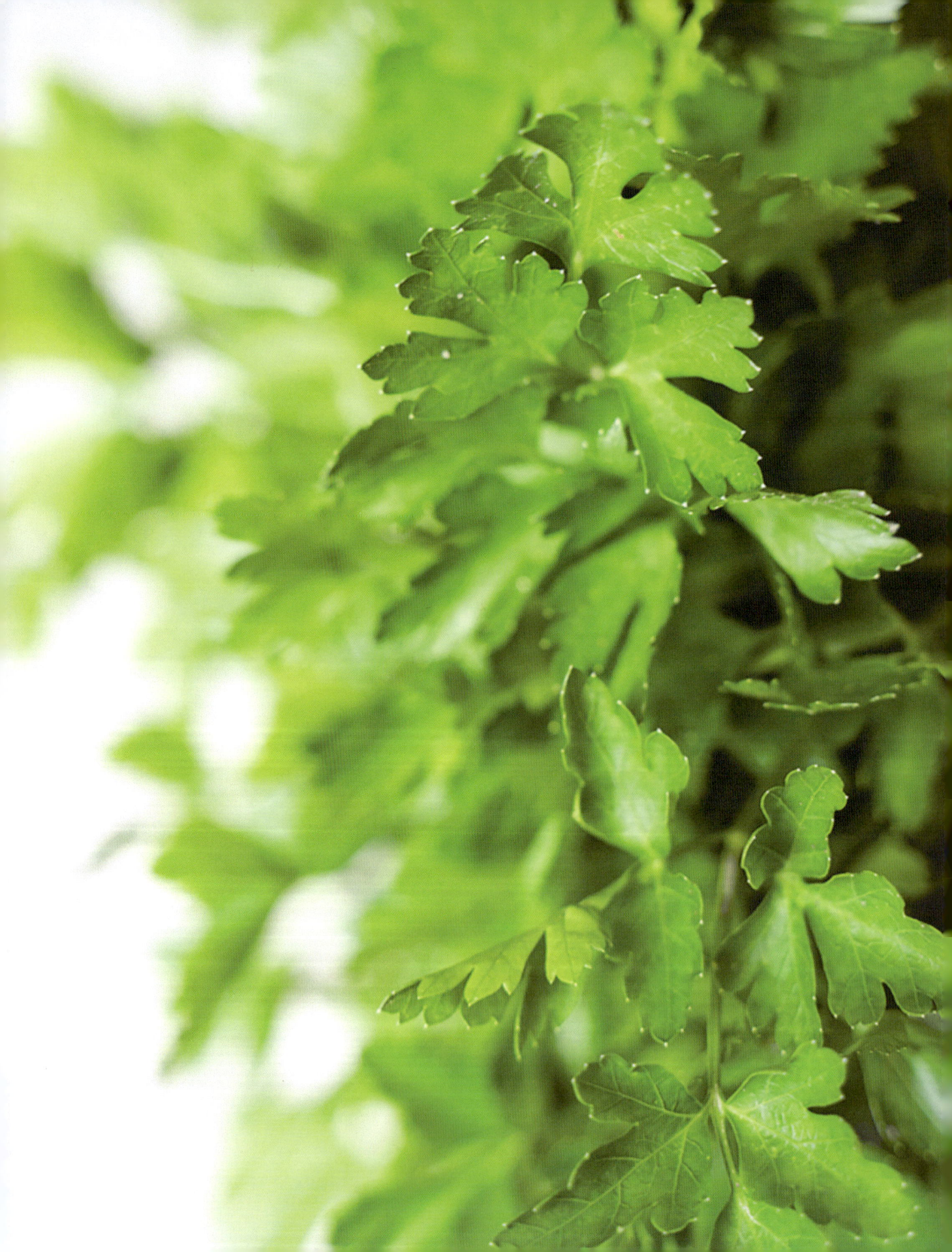

SWAP OUT & REMOVE

Begin to swap out and gradually **remove** the items listed below from your eating habits:

- Wheat
- Gluten-containing grains & oats
- Soy or soya products
- Quinoa
- Corn
- Legumes and beans
- Cows dairy products
- Margarine & Crisco
- Alcohol
- Coffee
- Tap water
- Non pasture-raised/grass-fed meat
- Non free-range or organic eggs
- Commercially farmed fish or seafood
- Processed and deep fried food
- Polyunsaturated oils (vegetable & seed oils)

Artificial ingredients and additives such as:

- High fructose corn syrup
- Sweeteners like aspartame, stevia and sucralose
- MSG
- Food colourings
- Preservatives
- Gums (such as guar gum)

SWAP IN & REPLACE

Gradually begin to **replace** the items you removed with the items below:

- Wheat-free bread & foods
- Gluten-free rice or coconut flour
- Gluten-free oats
- Rice puffs or flakes
- Lard, suet or ghee
- Olive oil or coconut oil
- Root vegetables
- Organic, grass-fed dairy goat products
- Organic, grass-fed/pasture-raised meat, organs and eggs (not fed any grains, soy or corn)
- Fresh or frozen fish
- Honey or maple syrup
- Bone broths and organic soups
- Good quality 90% dark chocolate
- Organic or frozen fruit and berries
- Filtered or still mineral water
- Coconut water
- Herbal or fruit teas like rooibos/red bush
- Coconut milk

"We all eat, and it would be a sad waste of opportunity to eat badly."

- ANNA THOMAS

"There is no sincerer love than the love of food."

– GEORGE BERNARD SHAW

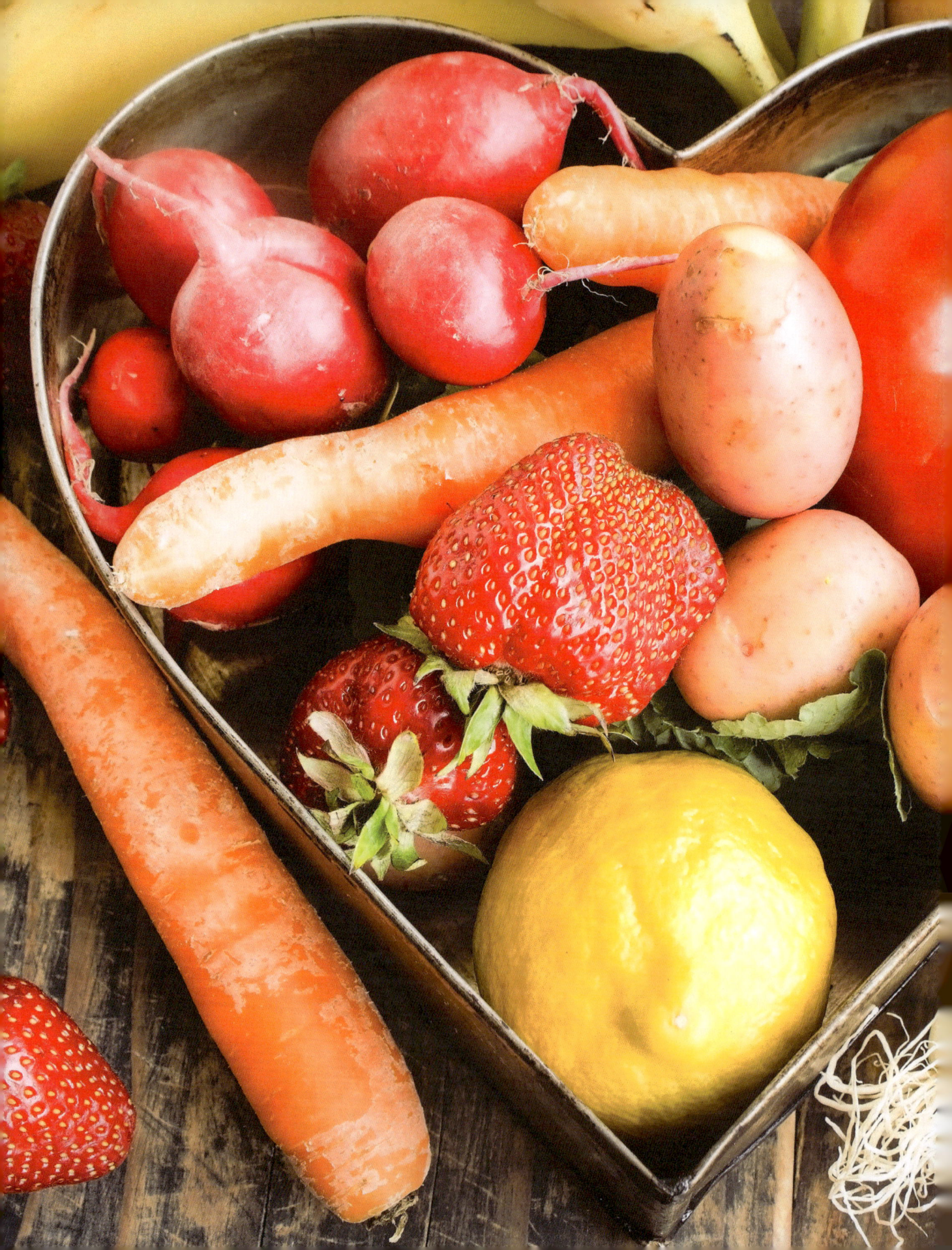

HOW FOOD IS 'MADE' IN OUR MODERN WORLD

In addition to the suggestions above, try to aim for all of the produce that you consume to fall under some, and ultimately all, of the below categories:

Organic

The requirements for food to be termed as organic can vary between countries and certifiers. However, generally, organic produce must have been grown or raised without genetic modification (GM), GM feed, man-made chemicals (such as fertilizers), growth regulators, feed additives, and irradiation. Organic products are also not allowed to contain any artificial colorings and sweeteners.

Do note that, although organic animal products are better than their non-organic counterparts, organically-raised animals are not always grass-fed or pasture-raised; after all, their feed just has to be organic. So, many cows, for example, can still be fed a non-grass diet and be classified as organic. That is why you should always strive for your produce to be organic and grass-fed/pasture-raised. Ideally, get to know your local butcher and visit the Farmer's Market. Become interested in how your food is made.

Grass-Fed or Pasture-Raised

Try to ensure that any beef, lamb and goat (and any of their organs or dairy) you consume are grass-fed. For eggs, chicken and pork (and any of their organs) you are looking for pasture-fed. Grass-fed or pasture-raised set-ups provide the best diet for their respective animals and offer a far better quality of life. Such factors will be reflected in the quality and nutrients of the meat, organs or other products and, of course, your body.

What If I Cannot Access These Products?

Sometimes it may not be possible to access pasture-raised eggs, chicken and pork. In such situations, the next best alternative then is free-range. However, always try to ensure you are buying pasture-raised as this makes a big difference on the quality and nutrients of the animal product.

If organic, grass-fed or pasture raised is not available or is over your budget then don't worry too much. You will still get lots of benefit from the whole food products compared to processed food. If possible try and ensure that the produce is still local and from small farms rather than big factory farms. If you are unsure about the quality of meat you are buying, then opt for leaner cuts. For fruit and vegetables, if you are unsure of the quality then ensure to peel them (if they have skins) before eating or cooking.

SHOPPING LIST

Here is an ideal shopping list to help you get started but bear in mind that this is not a comprehensive list. Also, some items may not be available in supermarkets so be sure to check out farmer's markets, local health food stores, local butchers, local fishmongers, and local green grocers. If necessary, you can also go online and see if there are relatively local suppliers or farmers that deliver to you.

It can be a good idea to get to know your local butcher or greengrocer to find out what they feed their animals or spray on their crops.

Please ensure that your produce is fresh, high quality, organic, pasture-raised, natural, seed oil free, etc. All of the produce listed below has been recommended on the assumption that you are buying the best quality, most natural forms of it (as advised on page 21).

Vegetables

Leaves*
Kale*
Spinach
Collard greens
Swiss chard
Rocket
Lettuce
Radicchio
Bok choy
Brussels sprouts
Watercress

Bulbs
Leek
Shallot
Onion
Spring onion
Garlic*

Roots
Beetroot
Carrot
Celeriac
Parsnip
Radish
Swede
Turnip

Fruits
Courgette
Cucumber
Aubergine
Plantain
Pumpkin
Chilli*
Squash
Avocado
Tomato
Pepper

Stems
Celery*
Asparagus
Rhubarb

Tubers
White potato
Sweet potato
Yam
Artichokes

Flowers
Cauliflower
Broccoli
Choi sum

Mushrooms
Portobello
Shiitake

Fruits

Pome
Pears
Apples

Tropical
Pineapples
Papayas
Mangoes
Kiwifruit
Guavas
Passionfruit
Coconuts

Citrus
Oranges
Tangerines
Lemons
Limes
Grapefruit

Berries
Strawberries
Blackberries
Blueberries
Raspberries
Goji berries
Grapes
Cranberries

Stone
Cherries
Olives
Apricots
Peaches
Plums
Nectarines

Melons
Watermelon
Cantaloupe
Honeydew

Grains*

White rice
Brown rice
Gluten-free oats
   (always soaked
   or cooked)

Oils & Butters

Coconut oil
Olive oil
Butter
Suet
Ghee
Lard
Tallow

Condiments

Kimchi
Vinegar (e.g. balsamic)
Mustard
Ketchup
Organic sauerkraut
Worcestershire sauce

Milks

Coconut milk
Rice milk
Goat's milk

Seafood

Salmon
Cod
Haddock
Trout
Mackerel
Herring
Sardines
Tuna
Lobster
Crab
Oysters
Scallops

Meat

Beef
Pork
Lamb
Venison
Veal
Duck
Turkey
Chicken

Organs & Parts

Liver
Tongue
Heart
Sweetbread
Tripe
Bone marrow
Gelatin powder
Collagen powder

Animal Products

Cheese
Cream
Eggs
Yoghurt
Royal jelly
Bee pollen

Beverages

Rooibos redbush tea
Fruit teas
Herbal teas
Coconut water
Fresh, pure fruit juice
Still mineral water

Sweets

Unpasteurized honey
Maple syrup
Raw honeycomb
Agar nectar
Jam
Marmalade

Baking items

Coconut flour
Rice flour
Vanilla extract
Baking powder
Baking soda

Other

Rice protein
Pea protein
Spirulina
Chorella

*Be careful with these foods. Sometimes they do not agree with certain women with endometriosis. Eliminate initially and then introduce slowly to see how your body responds.

In any recipes that use dairy products, it is recommend to use coconut or goat substitutes to begin with. If you do use dairy products always opt for full fat versions. And of course make it organic and grass-fed (and raw if possible)!

Please note that all foods listed in the following recipes are a reflection of what has been discussed in previous pages. For example, eggs are referring to pasture-raised, organic eggs.

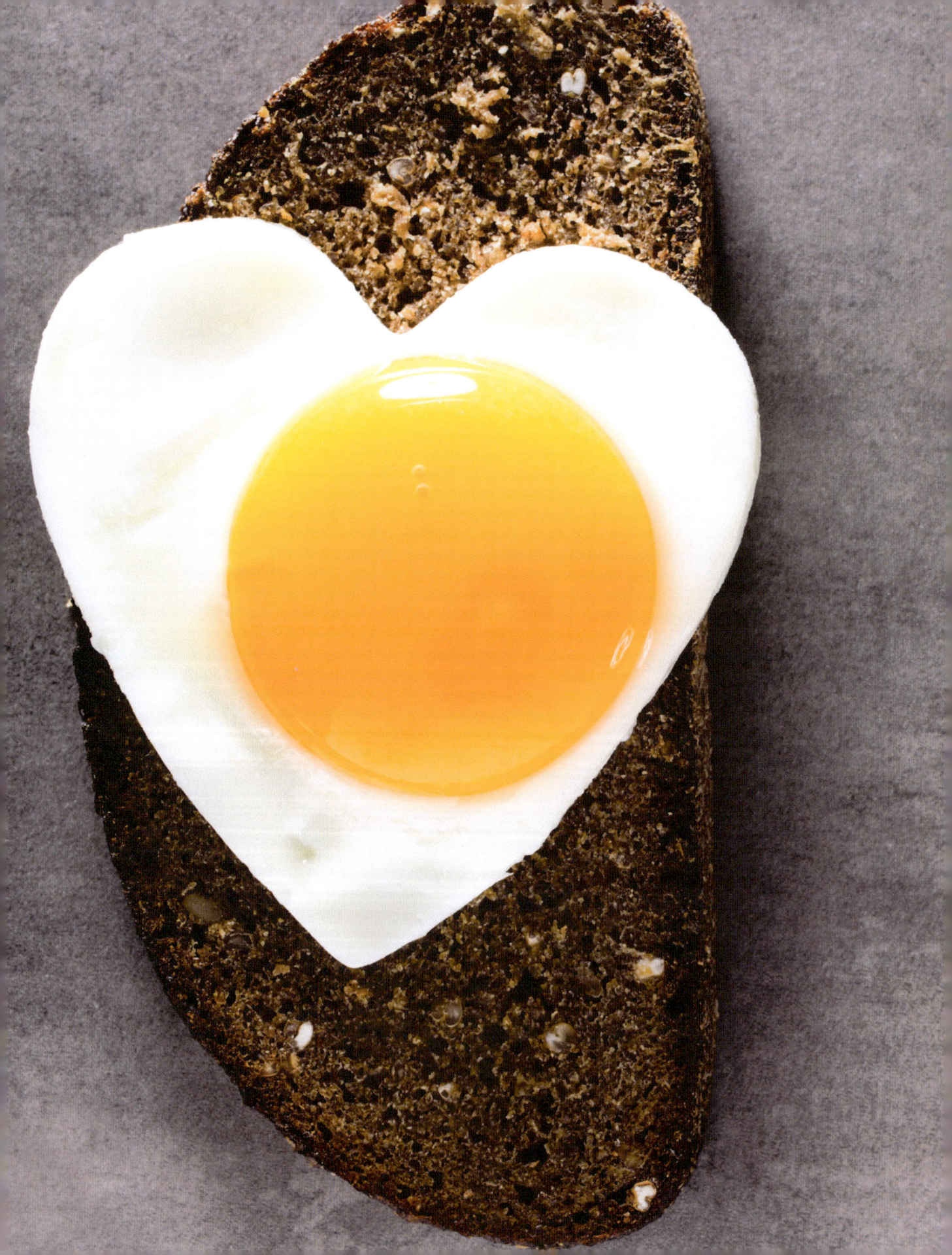

BREAKFAST LIKE A QUEEN!

There's an old saying I have adapted. *"Breakfast like a queen; lunch like a princess; dinner like a pauper."*

Breakfast is the most important meal of the day as it "breaks" the fast of the night.

The body uses a lot of energy stores for growth and repair of cells throughout the night, so always try to eat within one hour of waking to boost your energy levels and alertness for the day ahead.

Remember you cannot run your body on an empty stomach. You need to fill up your body as you would fill up the tank of a car with petrol.

Running on an empty stomach can lead to a release of stress hormones such as cortisol and adrenaline so that your body can mobilise fat stores and catabolise muscle so that it can get the energy it needs. This may add great stress and imbalance to an already inflamed body.

If you are not a morning person and struggle to eat solid food first thing, then consider "drinking" your breakfast instead.

I recommend to our Endobosses to start their day with a 'Power Shake'. The ingredients consist of organic rice and/or pea protein powder mixed with multi-vitamin powder in water. Having this, in addition to your breakfast meal, gives your body the essential extra nutrition it needs for the ultimate start to your day.

> *"Probably one of the most private things in the world is an egg until it is broken."*
>
> — MFK FISHER

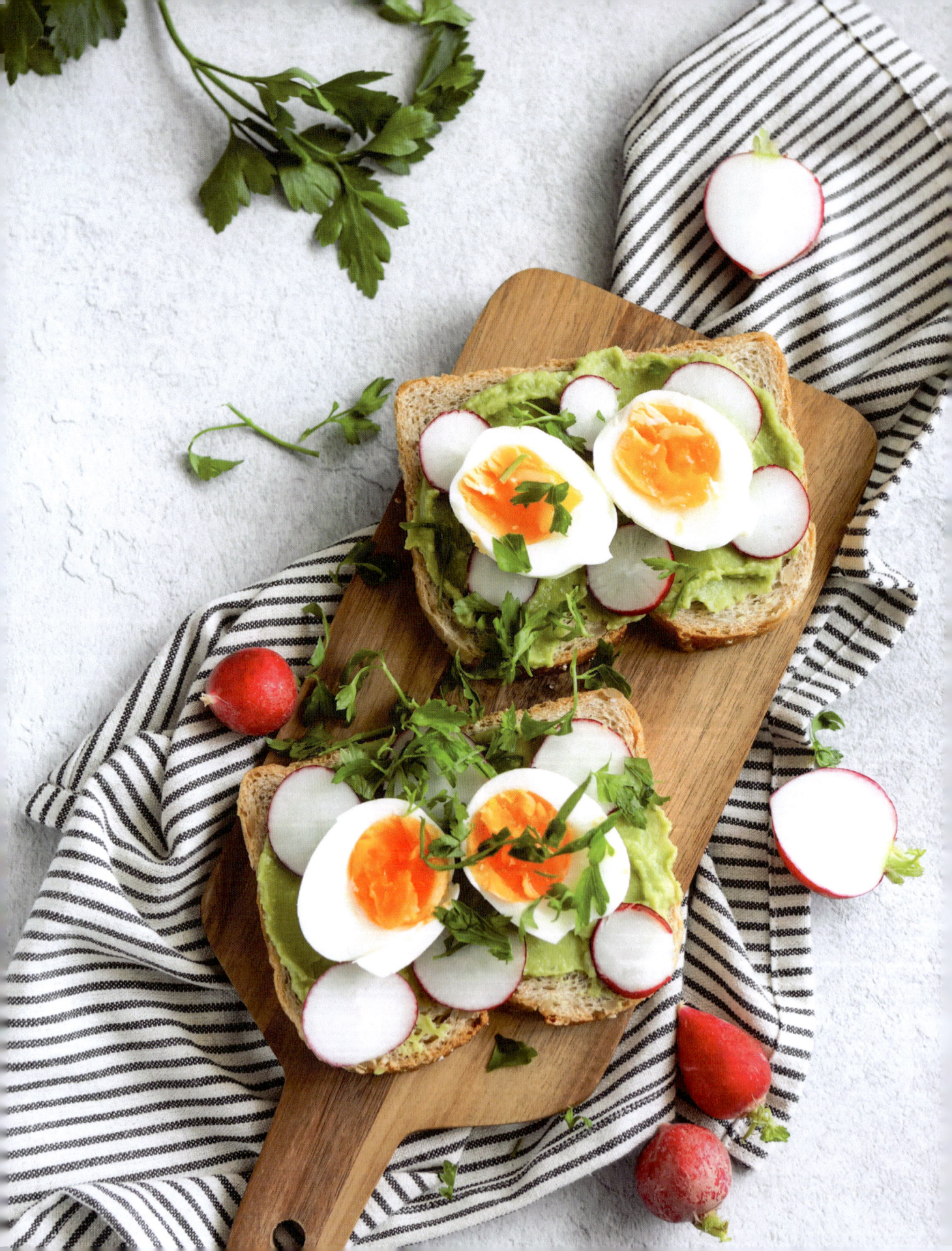

CODDLED EGGS

INGREDIENTS:

Eggs (with shell intact)

METHOD:

- Fill a pot with enough water to submerge an egg and bring it to the boil.
- Bring down the heat so the water comes from a rolling boil to a rapid simmer. Using a slotted serving spoon, gently place your eggs in the water, being careful not to crack them. Start a timer or keep a note of the time.
- The length of time you boil your egg depends on how you like your yolk, where ever that is between runny or cooked. However, I do recommend a runny yolk as it is far more nutritious than a cooked one. Below is a rough guide on how to achieve your desired yolk:
  - Soft boiled: 5 minutes
  - Soft-hard boiled: 7 minutes
  - Hard boiled: 9 minutes
- Once your egg has been boiling for the desired amount of time, remove the pan from the heat and plunge the eggs into cold water.
- When they have slightly cooled, remove the eggs from the water and either serve as they are, or peel the shell away.

Eggs are great to have on the go and a handy snack later in the day. Enjoy your eggs alongside some of our other recipes, or with cooked meat or cheese. Sprinkle some salt over your egg for more flavour!

"Go To Work On An Egg"

- UNITED KINGDOM'S EGG MARKETING BOARD DURING 1950S AND 1960S

SCRAMBLED EGGS

INGREDIENTS:

Eggs
Butter-5g per egg
Salt (to taste)
Lemon juice (optional)

METHOD:

- Break the eggs into a bowl, add in the salt and beat well until combined.

- *Optional:* add a drop of lemon juice per egg. Acid helps eggs not lose as much water when being cooked. The result is eggs that are even more moist and creamy!

- Pour the eggs into a pan and add in the corresponding amount of butter.

- Then, place the pan on a cooker and turn on the heat but only to a low temperature. This is important as if cooked at too high a heat, the eggs will dry out; this is what has happened when you are served scrambled eggs with a pool of liquid beneath.

- Using a spatula, stir the eggs constantly. Gradually, the butter will melt as the eggs heat up. Keep stirring and be patient. It may take a little while for eggs to start to come together.

- When they do, keep stirring and only when they are just about to reach the desired consistency, then remove from the heat and serve.

"Don't put all your eggs in one basket."

– JULIA CHILD

TROPICAL FRUIT SALAD   Serves 2

INGREDIENTS:

1 cup mixed berries

1 cup sliced banana

1 cup sliced kiwi

1/2 cup chopped pineapple

1/2 cup chopped apple

1 lime, juiced

2 tbsp honey

Salt (to taste)

METHOD:

- Mix the honey and lime juice in a small bowl. Add a pinch of salt.

- In a large bowl, combine all of the fruit. Pour the lime mixture over the mix and let it stand in the refrigerator for at least 20 minutes.

- Remove from the refrigerator when ready to eat. Sprinkle with more salt if needed. Enjoy!

> "Don't eat anything your Great-Grandmother wouldn't recognise as food."
>
> – MICHAEL POLLAN

PLUM BREAKFAST CAKE — Serves 8

INGREDIENTS:

1 cup coconut flour
2 tbsp rice flour
2 tsp baking powder
2 tsp vanilla extract
2 tbsp coconut oil
4 tbsp honey

2 eggs
3 tsp gelatin powder
1/3 cup plums, destoned, mashed
1 tsp cinnamon
Salt (to taste)

METHOD:

- In a mixing bowl, combine together coconut flour, rice flour, baking soda and vanilla extract. Add the eggs, coconut oil, salt and half the honey. Whisk together until a smooth, dough-like mixture then set aside.

- In another bowl, combine the mashed plums, salt, honey and cinnamon.

- Transfer the dough mixture onto a baking sheet and roll it into a long shape that can be divided into six equal rectangles.

- Next, create small 1.5cm/2cm tall rectangles and create 2 small wells adjacent to each other within the dough and dollop with the plum mixture. Place in the refrigerator for approximately 20 minutes before baking.

- Meanwhile, preheat the oven to 180°C. Once ready, bake the pieces for approximately 15-20 minutes, or until a nice golden color.

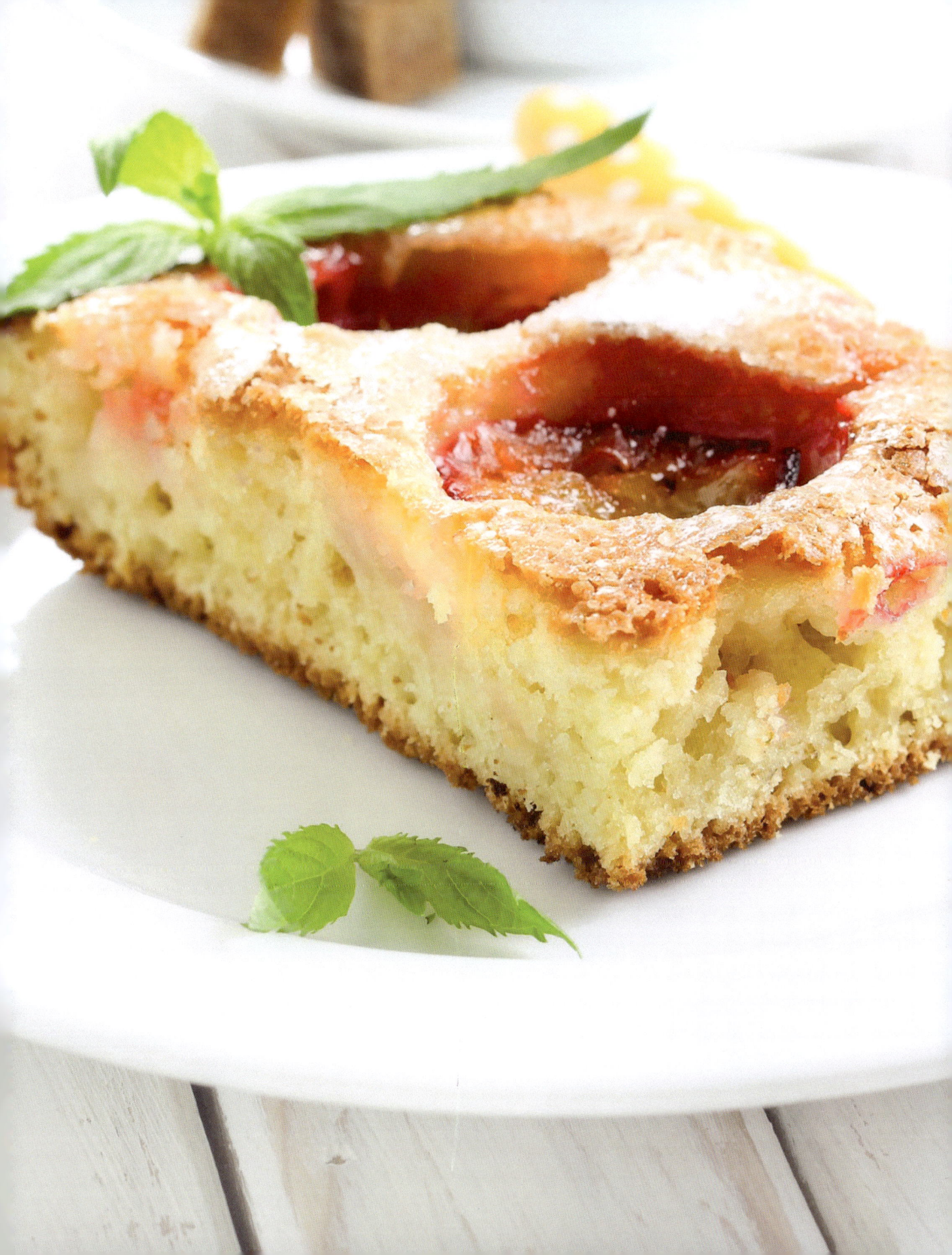

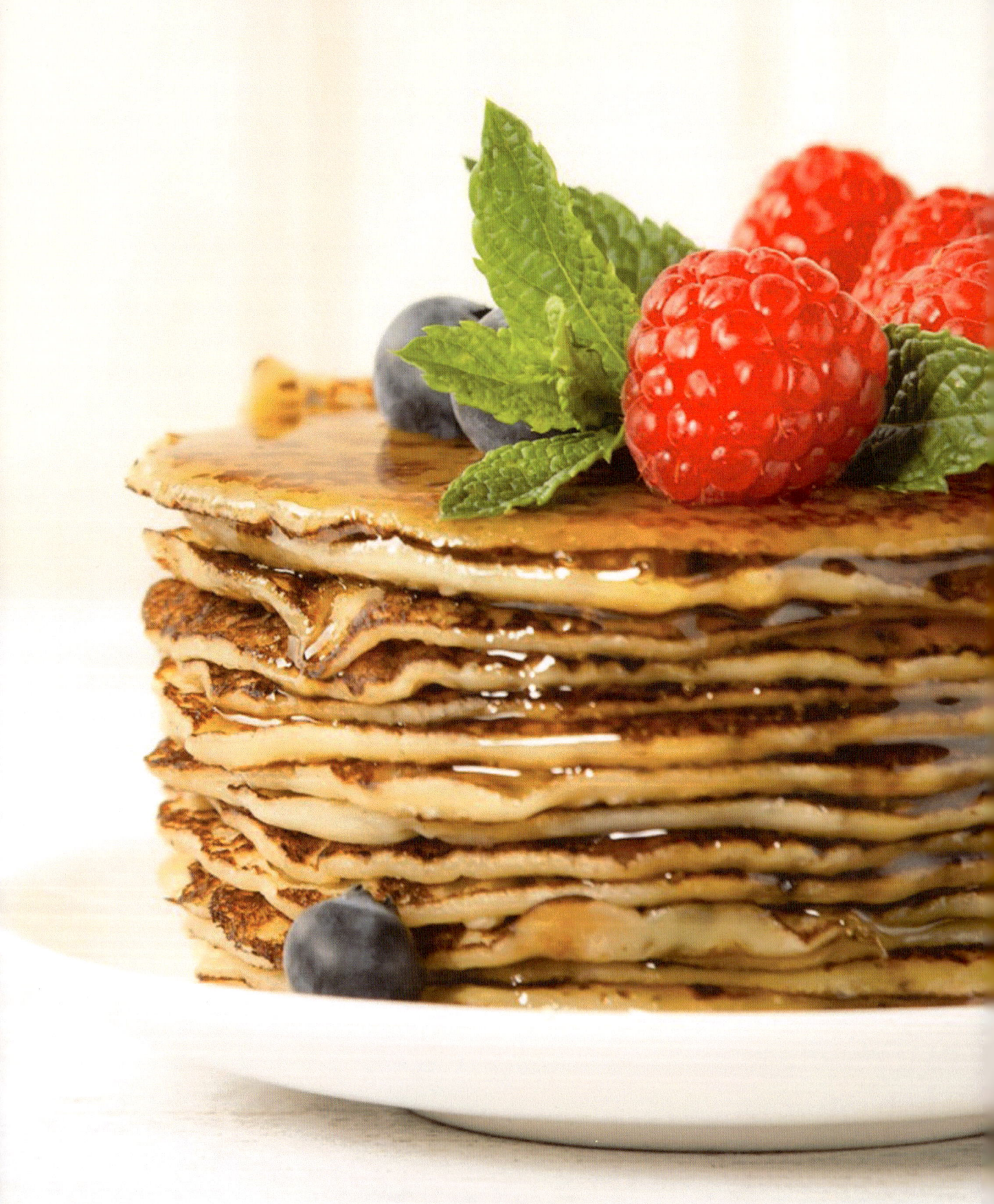

PERFECT GRIDDLECAKES   Serves 4

INGREDIENTS:

1 cup rice flour

2 eggs

1 tsp gelatin powder

1 tsp baking powder

1 cup milk

2 tbsp honey

1 tsp butter

Salt (to taste)

METHOD:

- Put all the ingredients in the bowl and mix thoroughly. Heat a pan on a medium heat with some butter.

- Spoon some of the batter into the pan. When bubbles can be seen to rise to the surface, flip the griddle cake over. Once the second side is browned, lift off the pan and place to one side.

- Repeat until all the batter is used. Enjoy!

(*You can enjoy these on their own but I recommend serving with the scrambled egg recipe or the banana delight recipe. Equally, these work great with some classic jam and butter).

BANANA LOAF BREAD — Serves 6

INGREDIENTS

3 very ripe bananas, peeled, mashed
2 cups rice flour
2 eggs
1/3 cup butter
1 tsp baking powder
2 tsp gelatin powder
1 tsp vanilla extract
2 tbsp honey
Salt (to taste)

METHOD

- Preheat the oven to 180°C.

- Add the butter, eggs, bananas in a bowl and mix whilst adding in the honey and vanilla extract together. Add some salt.

- Mix well until light and fluffy. Gently fold in the flour, gelatin and baking powder until a smooth consistency.

- Butter a loaf tin and line with baking paper. Then, pour the mixture into the tin.

- Transfer to the oven and bake for 45 minutes or until it is well-risen and golden-brown.

- Remove from the oven and check the center is cooked at intervals by gently pushing a knife or skewer into the bread and drawing it out; if you see wet batter or overly soft crumbs then it needs longer. Do this a few times. Also, ensure you are pushing straight down and up without letting the knife move side to side.

- When ready, leave to cool in the tin for a few minutes, then place onto a wire rack to cool completely before serving.

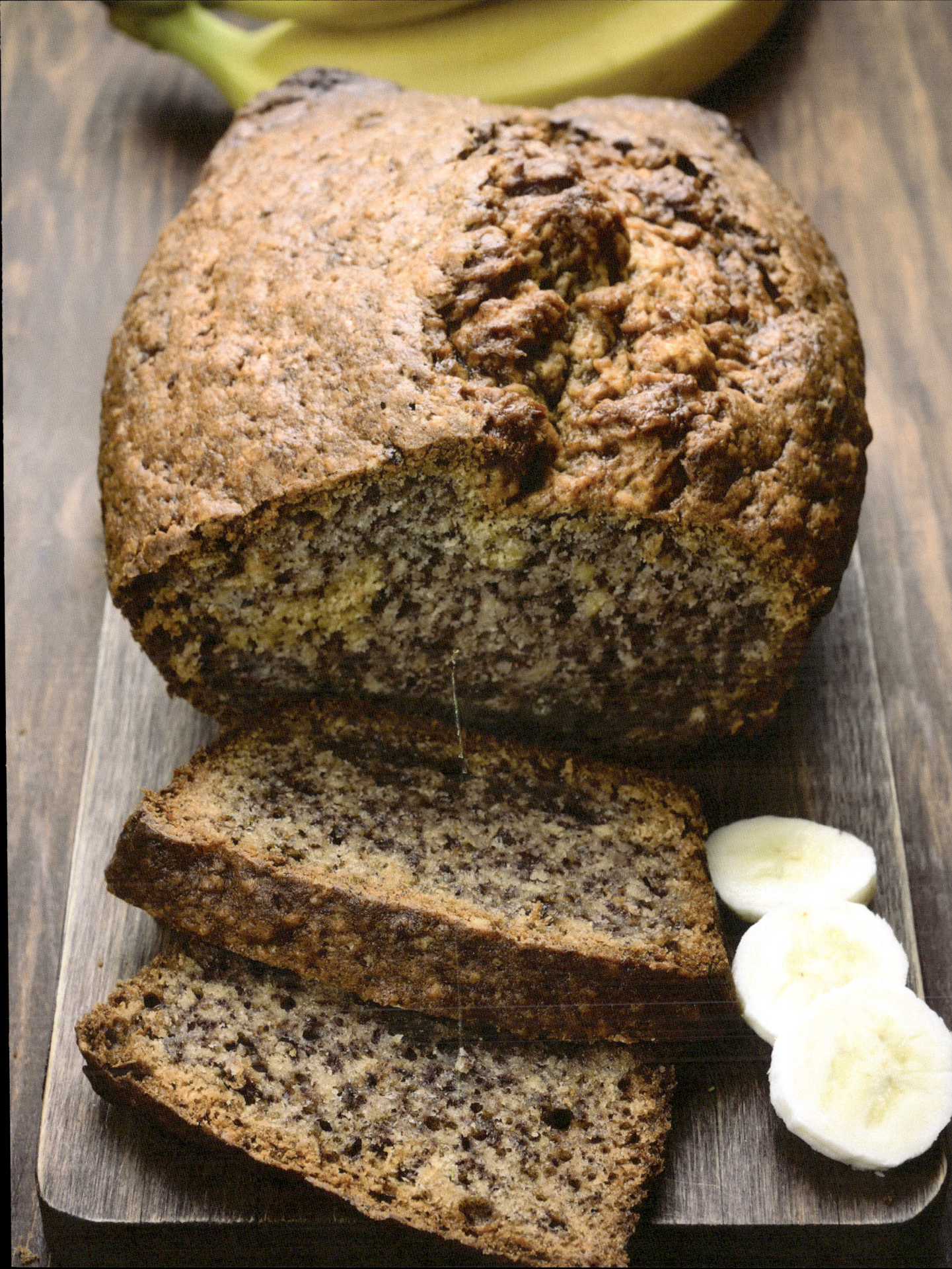

"First we eat, then we do everything else."

—M.F.K. FISHER

BLUE BANANA DELIGHT   Serves 1-2

INGREDIENTS:

3 bananas
1 cup blueberries
4 egg yolks
1 cup coconut milk
1/2 cup yoghurt

3 tbsp honey
1 tsp vanilla extract
Salt (to taste)

METHOD:

- Peel the bananas and break into chunks.
- Combine with all other ingredients into a blender and mix until a smooth paste forms.
- Serve immediately, or keep in the refrigerator to thicken the mixture. Serve cold.

(*For an extra protein boost add a scoop of organic vanilla rice protein powder and with some extra coconut milk to keep the consistency).

SPINACH & BACON OMELETTE   Serves 2

INGREDIENTS:

1/2 cup chopped spinach
2 rashers dry cured bacon
6 eggs
1 tsp butter, for frying
1 tsp fresh parsley, chopped
Salt (to taste)

METHOD:

- Heat up a pan over a low-medium temperature. Once warmed, add the butter and then the bacon. Remove the bacon from the pan once cooked and add in the spinach.

- Gently cook in the butter and bacon fat until almost wilted. Set aside with the bacon when done.

- Remove the pan from the heat for the time being.

- Next, whisk up the eggs and some salt. Break up the spinach and bacon into small chunks and add to the mixture.

- Reheat the pan, and pour the mixture in.

- As the eggs start to set, flip the omelette over.

- When ready, transfer the omelette to a plate and sprinkle and serve with the parsley.

AUTUMN COMFORT FOOD

Inspired by **EndoBoss® Beginner** – Natalie Krier from USA

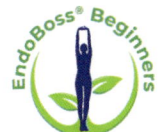

Serves 4

INGREDIENTS:

- 1 butternut squash, peeled, deseeded, cubed
- 6 eggs
- 8 bacon rashers
- 2 ripe avocados, peeled, pitted, cubed
- 3 tbsp coconut oil
- Pepper (to taste)
- Salt (to taste)

METHOD:

- Preheat the oven to 200°C. Place the squash on an oven tray with 1 tbsp coconut oil and some salt. Roast until soft and slightly golden (about 25 minutes).

- Place the bacon on an oven tray grill and cook until crispy. When done, break up into smaller pieces and set aside.

- Meanwhile, heat a frying pan with 1 tbsp coconut oil and fry the eggs, removing once the white is cooked but the yolk still runny. Add the other tbsp coconut oil if necessary.

- Finally, mix all the bacon, squash, avocado and eggs together in a big bowl. Break up the eggs into smaller bits during this process. Doing so will also release the yolk, making it like a sauce for the other ingredients.

- Taste and season with salt and pepper as desired. Serve immediately.

PERFECT PORRIDGE   Serves 2

INGREDIENTS:

4 cups coconut milk or water

2 tbsp honey

1 cup gluten-free oats

Cinnamon (to taste)

Salt (to taste)

METHOD:

- Place the oats, salt and milk in a pan. Place the pan on a high heat and start stirring the mixture.

- Once the mixture starts bubbling, turn down the heat slightly and continue to cook and stir for a further 5-10 minutes.

- When done, transfer the porridge to a bowl and top with the honey and cinnamon, or any other ingredients that you wish!

"Cooking well doesn't mean cooking fancy"

— JULIA CHILD

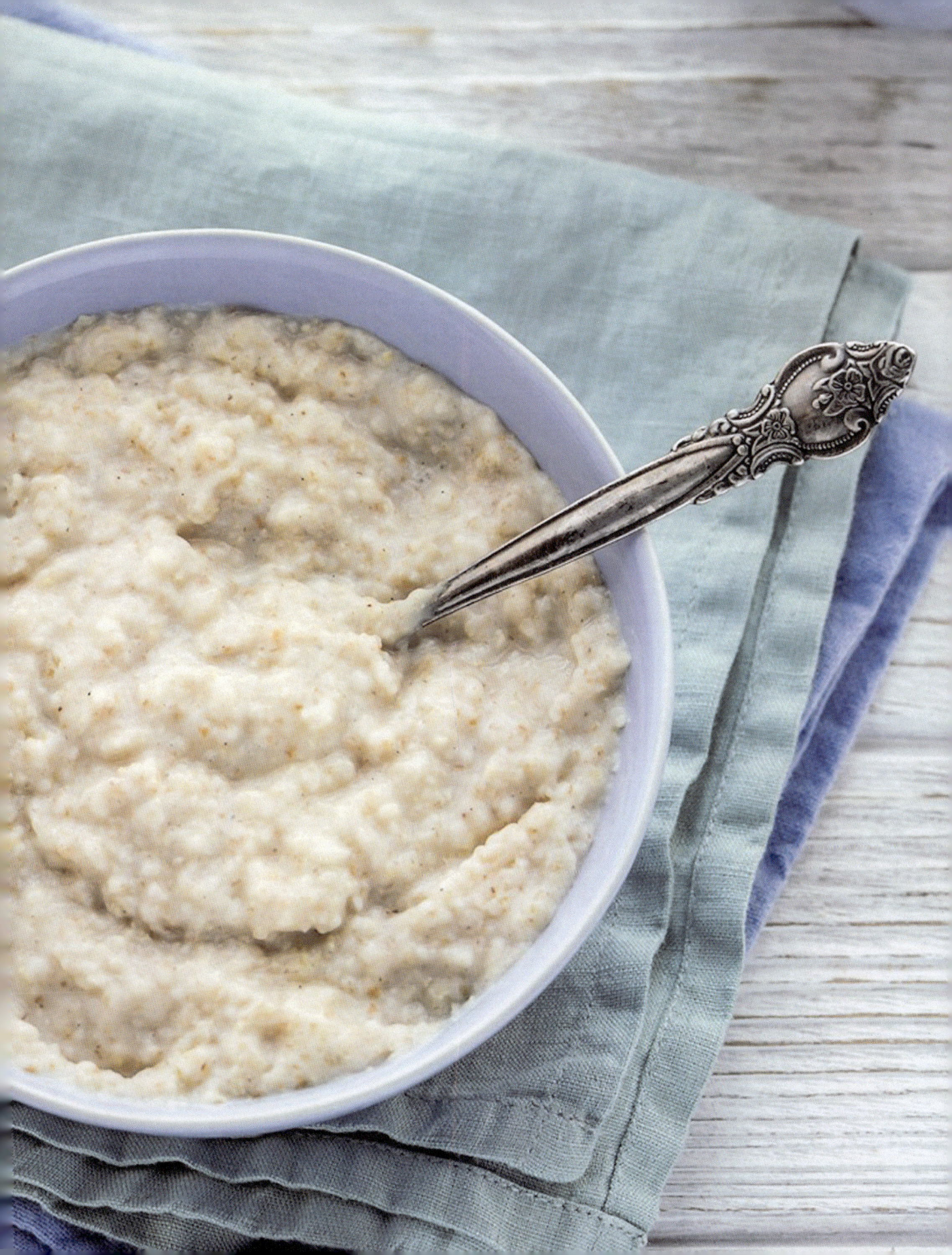

*"Why not go out on a limb?
Isn't that where the fruit is?"*

– FRANK SCULLY

INDULGENT PROTEIN YOGHURT   Serves 2

INGREDIENTS:

3 cups coconut yoghurt

3 tbsp raw honey

1/2 cup protein powder

1 tbsp bee pollen

2 tbsp dessicated coconut

1 cup fresh berries

Salt (to taste)

METHOD:

- Mix the yoghurt with the honey, protein powder, dessicated coconut and some salt.

- Divide between bowls and then top with the fresh berries and bee pollen. Add more toppings if you like.

- If the mixture is too thick for your liking then you can thin it with some coconut milk.

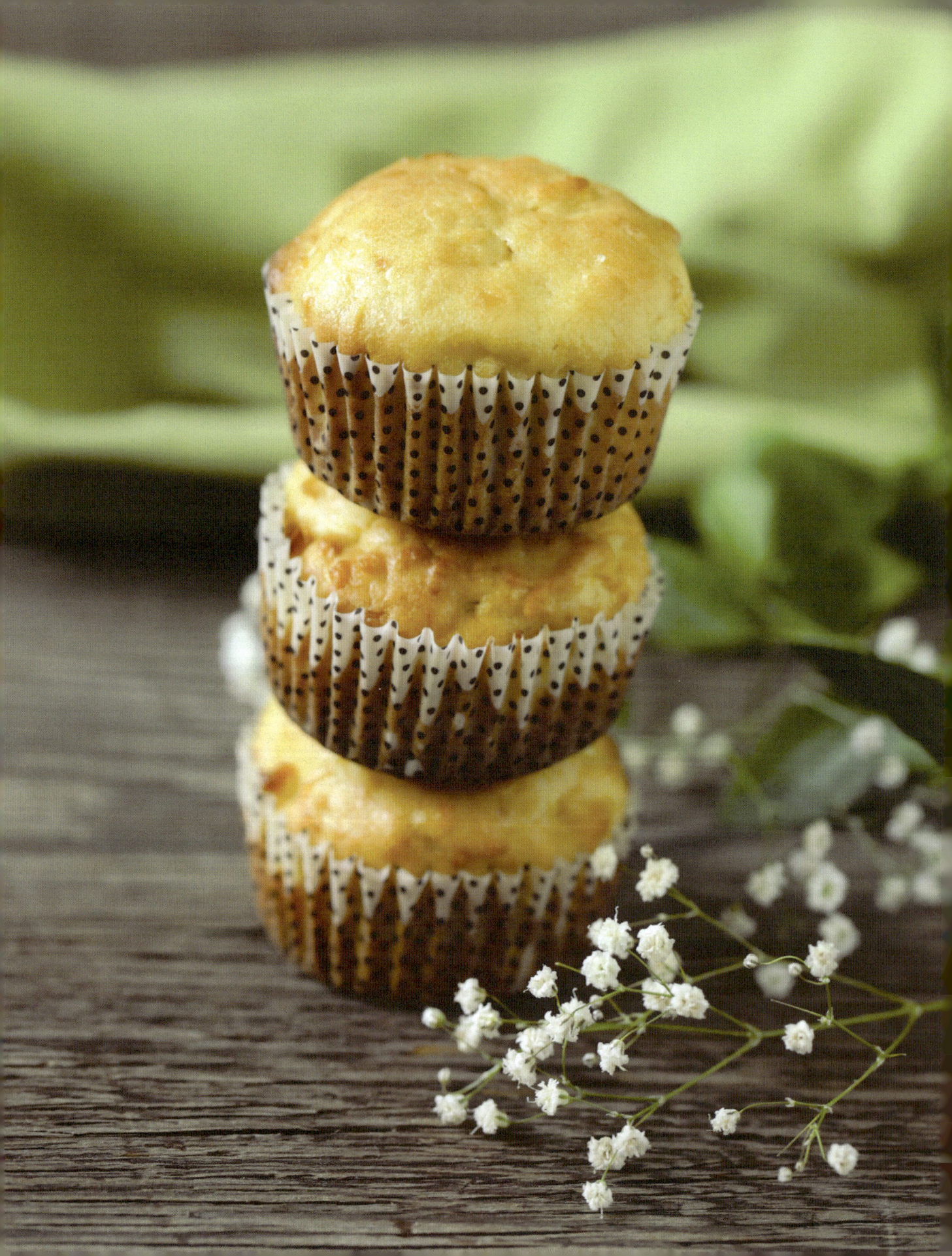

AVOCADO BREAKFAST MUFFINS   Serves 8

INGREDIENTS:

1 cup rice flour
2 cups coconut flour
4 tbsp honey
2 tsp baking powder
2 ripe avocados
2 eggs

1 tsp vanilla extract
1 tbsp coconut oil
1/2 cup butter
1/2 cup coconut milk
3 tsp gelatin powder
Salt (to taste)

METHOD:

- Preheat the oven to 200°C.
- In a large bowl, combine all the ingredients.
- Pour into greased muffin molds and bake for about 20 minutes, until browned on top.
- Remove from the oven and allow to cool before eating.

(*For an extra hearty breakfast with more protein, serve with the scrambled eggs recipe).

"All happiness depends on a leisurely breakfast."

—JOHN GUNTHER

LEAFY GREEN PANCAKES

Inspired by **EndoBoss® Alumni** - Anita Clohesy from Australia

Serves 2

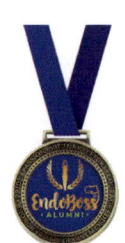

INGREDIENTS:

4 eggs
1 tbsp coconut oil
4 cups of leafy greens (e.g. spinach)
Salt (to taste)

METHOD:

- Blend the eggs and leafy greens together with some salt until smooth and frothy.
- Heat the coconut oil in a frying pan and then spoon some of the batter into the pan.
- Flip as bubbles start to form. Cook until lightly tanned on each side and then set aside.
- Repeat this until all the batter has been used.

(*Serve with some berries and lemon for a flavoursome twist or eat with some honey for a sweet kick).

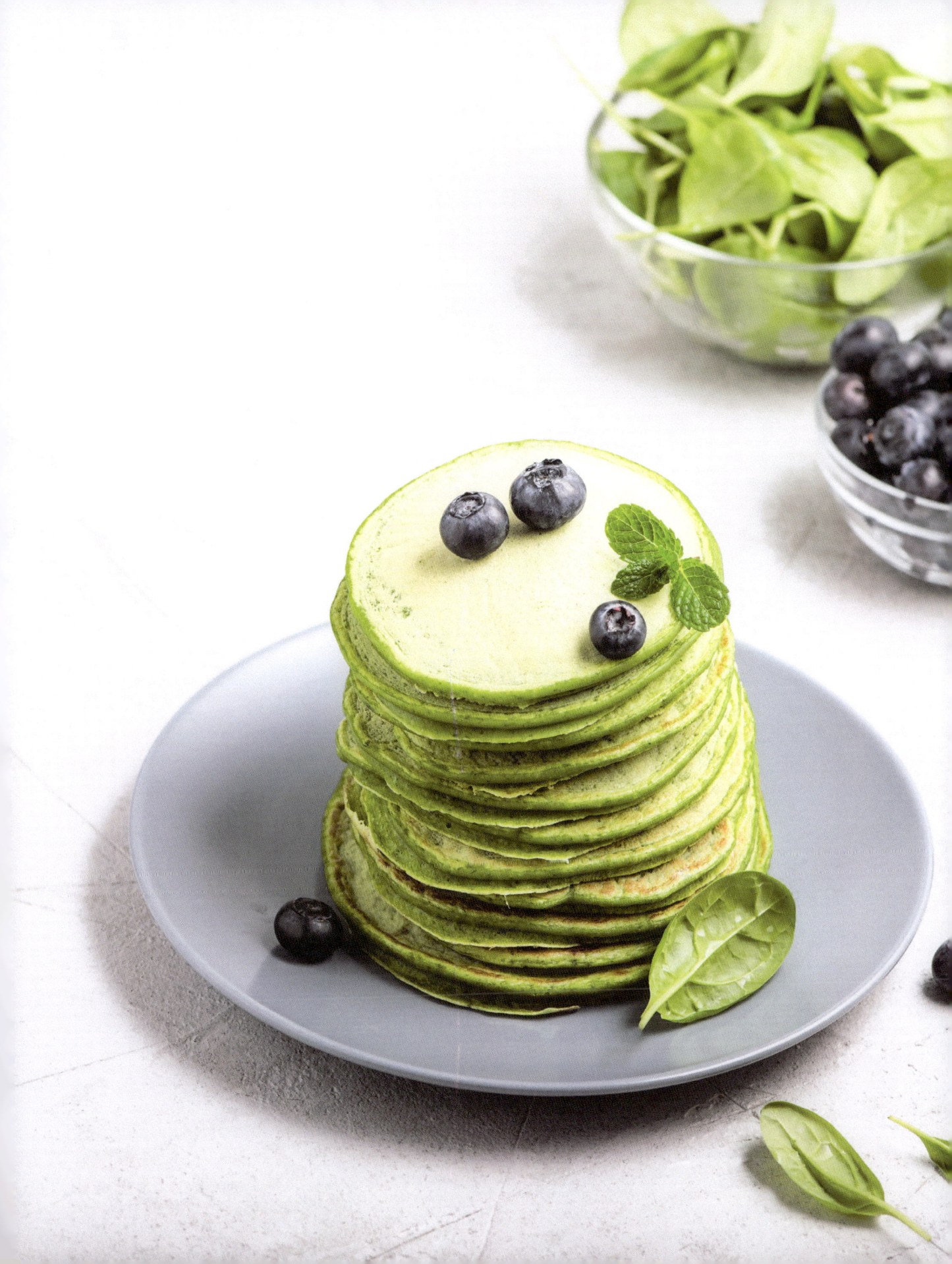

EGG & POTATO BREAKFAST WAFFLES Serves 4-6

INGREDIENTS:

1 pound of potatoes
4 eggs
1/2 small onion, finely diced
1/2 cup cheese
1/2 cup ham, diced
1 tbsp coconut oil
Paprika (to taste)
Pepper (to taste)
Salt (to taste)

METHOD:

- Preheat the oven to 180°C. Grate the potatoes and whisk the eggs. Place the grated potatoes in a sieve and wash through to remove excess starch. Squeeze any excess water from the potatoes by hand.

- Add the potatoes, eggs, oil, paprika, salt, pepper and onion to a bowl. Mix well and then transfer into a rectangular baking tray. Cook until the potatoes start to turn brown, approximately 15-20 minutes.

- Once the waffle base appears to be done, sprinkle the cheese and ham on top and place back in the oven for a few more minutes until the cheese is melted. Slice into squares, then serve and enjoy.

BAKED VEGETABLE FRITTATA — Serves 4-6

INGREDIENTS:

12 eggs
3 tbsp double cream
1 cup grated cheese
1 red onion, diced
1/4 cup spring onions, sliced
1 bell pepper, diced
1 cup spinach

1 garlic clove, minced
2 tbsp chives, chopped
1/2 cup mushrooms, chopped
1/2 cup cherry tomatoes, quartered
1 tbsp coconut oil
Salt (to taste)

METHOD:

- Preheat the oven to 180°C. Whisk the eggs, cheese, cream and some salt together in a bowl then set aside.
- Next, heat a pan with the oil and some salt.
- Add in the onion and pepper and cook for a few minutes before adding in the garlic, tomatoes and mushrooms.
- Cook for another few minutes and then mix in the spinach, cooking until the spinach has wilted and the other vegetables have begun to soften. Allow to cool.
- Then mix the eggs and vegetables together before transferring into an ovenproof dish.
- Cook in the oven for around 25 minutes until the mix has hardened but the centre still has a slight jiggle to it.
- Top with the chives and spring onions before slicing and serving.

FISHERMAN'S EGGS — Serves 4

INGREDIENTS:

1 cup tinned sardines, drained
1 large tomato, diced
3 garlic cloves, minced
1/4 cup parsley, chopped
1 red onion, diced
2 tbsp olives destoned
Pepper (to taste)
Salt (to taste)

METHOD:

- Preheat the oven to 180°C. Wash the sardines and mix with the parsley, onion, garlic, tomato, olives and some salt and pepper.
- Transfer the mix to an ovenproof dish and cook for 10 minutes.
- Once the time is up, crack the eggs on top of the other ingredients. Do this carefully to keep the yolks intact.
- Return to the oven for another 10-15 minutes until the whites have cooked.
- Remove from the oven and serve hot.

LIVER & ONIONS   Serves 6

INGREDIENTS:

1 pound sliced beef liver, cubed
1 large white onion, sliced
1 tbsp honey
2 tbsp butter
Pepper (to taste)
Salt (to taste)

METHOD:

- Place the butter in a frying pan and heat on a medium temperature.
- Briefly add the onions until they have softened a little and then remove.
- Turn up the heat a little and add the liver slices. Fry on one side until browned and flip.
- Now, add the onions back to the pan, along with some honey, salt and pepper.
- Keep cooking the liver until both sides are browned and there is only a small bit of pink left in the middle. Before turning off the heat, make sure the onions have fully softened.
- Serve hot and with the juices from the pan.

SOME ADDITIONAL SUPER, SIMPLE BREAKFAST IDEAS

- Rice puffs with coconut milk
- Bacon & fried eggs
- Sausages & poached eggs
- Yoghurt, fruit & honey
- Cold meats, cheese & fruit

You may wish to look at some of our lunch and dinner recipes as these too can be used for breakfast if you wish.

The following pages show some juices you can make which are a great breakfast addition.

Breakfast On The Move?

- Hard boiled eggs
- Coconut yoghurt pot
- Green juice & protein powder
- Beef or venison jerky with fresh orange
- Cured meat with a fruit pot
- Whole cucumber & small goats cheese block

Buy snacks that are organic or grass-fed. Be on the look out in the ingredients lists for seed oils or nasty additives. It is so important to plan ahead and order in or prepare high quality meals in advance especially if travelling.

Remember "If you fail to plan, you plan to fail."

SMOOTHIES & JUICES

"It's difficult to think anything but pleasant thoughts while eating a homegrown tomato."

—LEWIS GRIZZARD

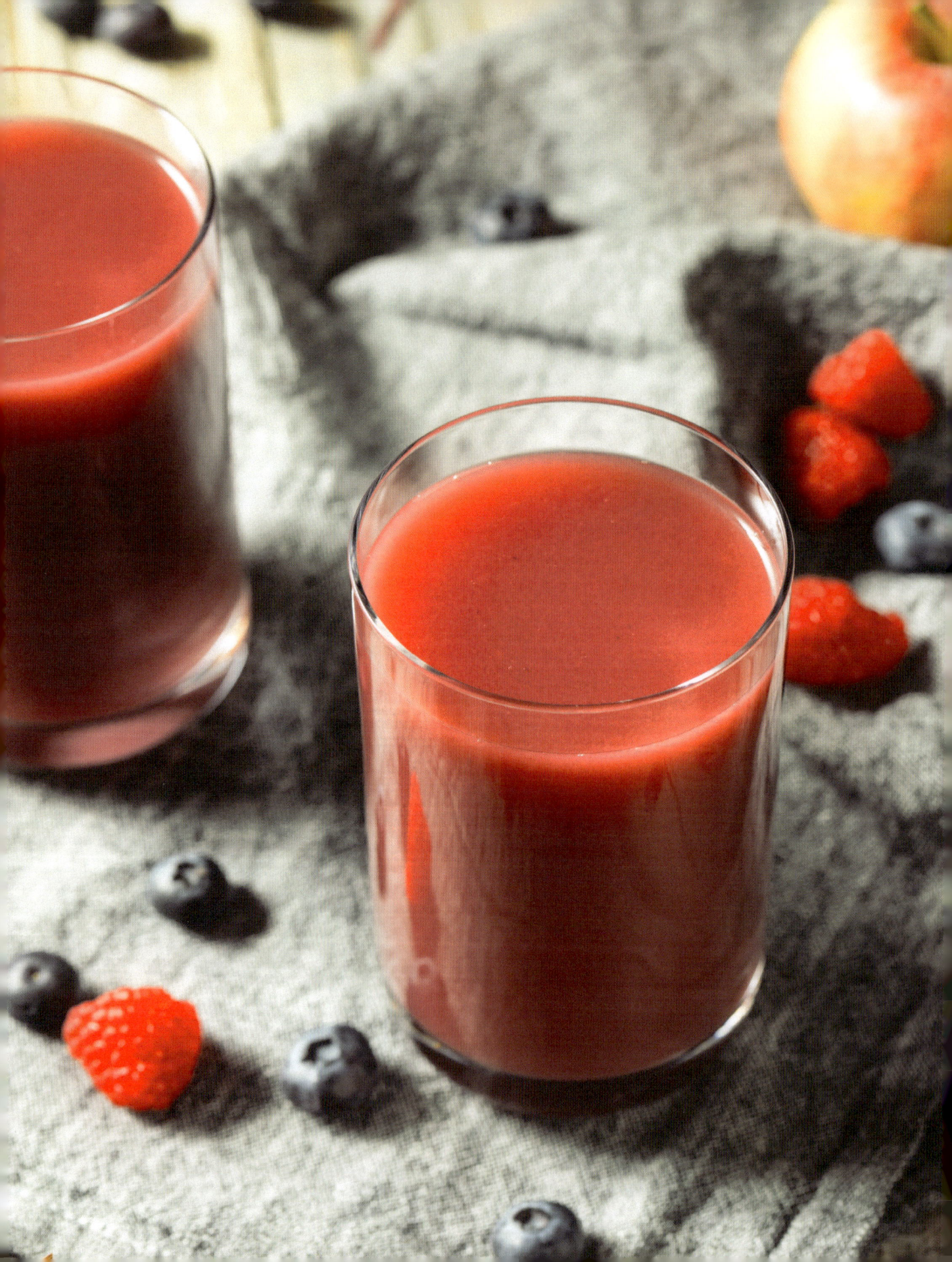

VITAMIN C FRUIT BLAST   Serves 1

INGREDIENTS:

4 oranges, peeled
1/2 cup blackcurrants
2 guavas, skinned
4 kiwis, peeled

METHOD:

- Combine the ingredients in a blender and mix for 30 seconds. Serve cold.
- Add some salt or honey for extra sweetness if desired.

OVERTLY ORANGE JUICE   Serves 1

INGREDIENTS:

8 carrots, ends chopped off
3 oranges, peeled
3 figs, skinned
1/2 mango, peeled and pitted
4 apricots, destoned

1 tbsp fresh ginger, skinned

METHOD:

- Add the ingredients to a juicer one at time and collect the juice in to a glass. Mix before drinking.
- Add some salt or honey for extra sweetness if desired.

JOLLY GREEN SMOOTHIE   Serves 1

INGREDIENTS:

1 ripe avocado, peeled, destoned
3 cups spinach
1/2 cup coconut milk
1/4 cup parsley

METHOD:

- Wash and drain the spinach.
- Combine all the ingredients into a blender and mix for about 30 seconds until smooth. Serve cold.
- Add some salt or honey for extra sweetness if desired.
- To make it extra nutritious consider adding in a tablespoon of protein powder when blending.

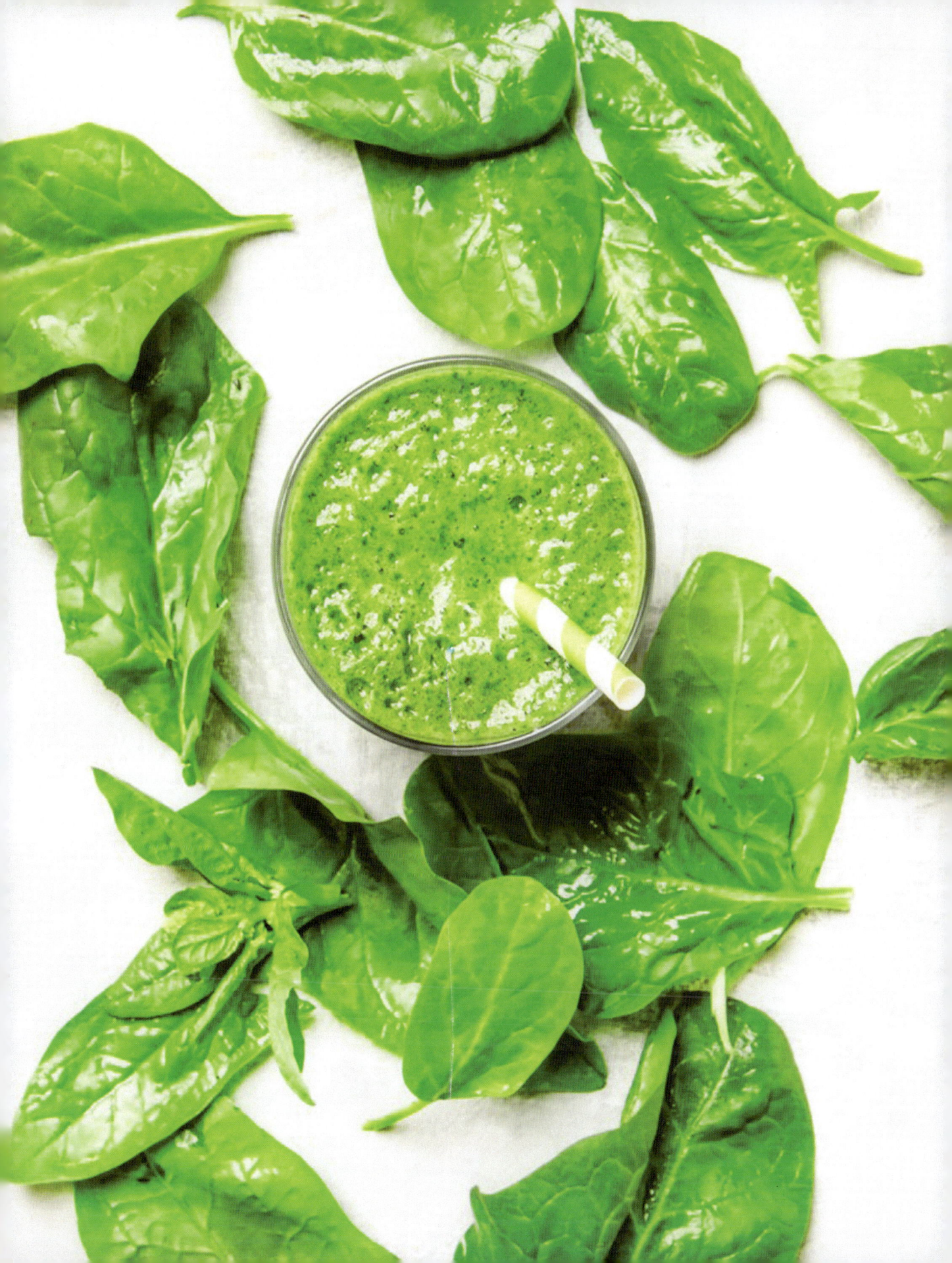

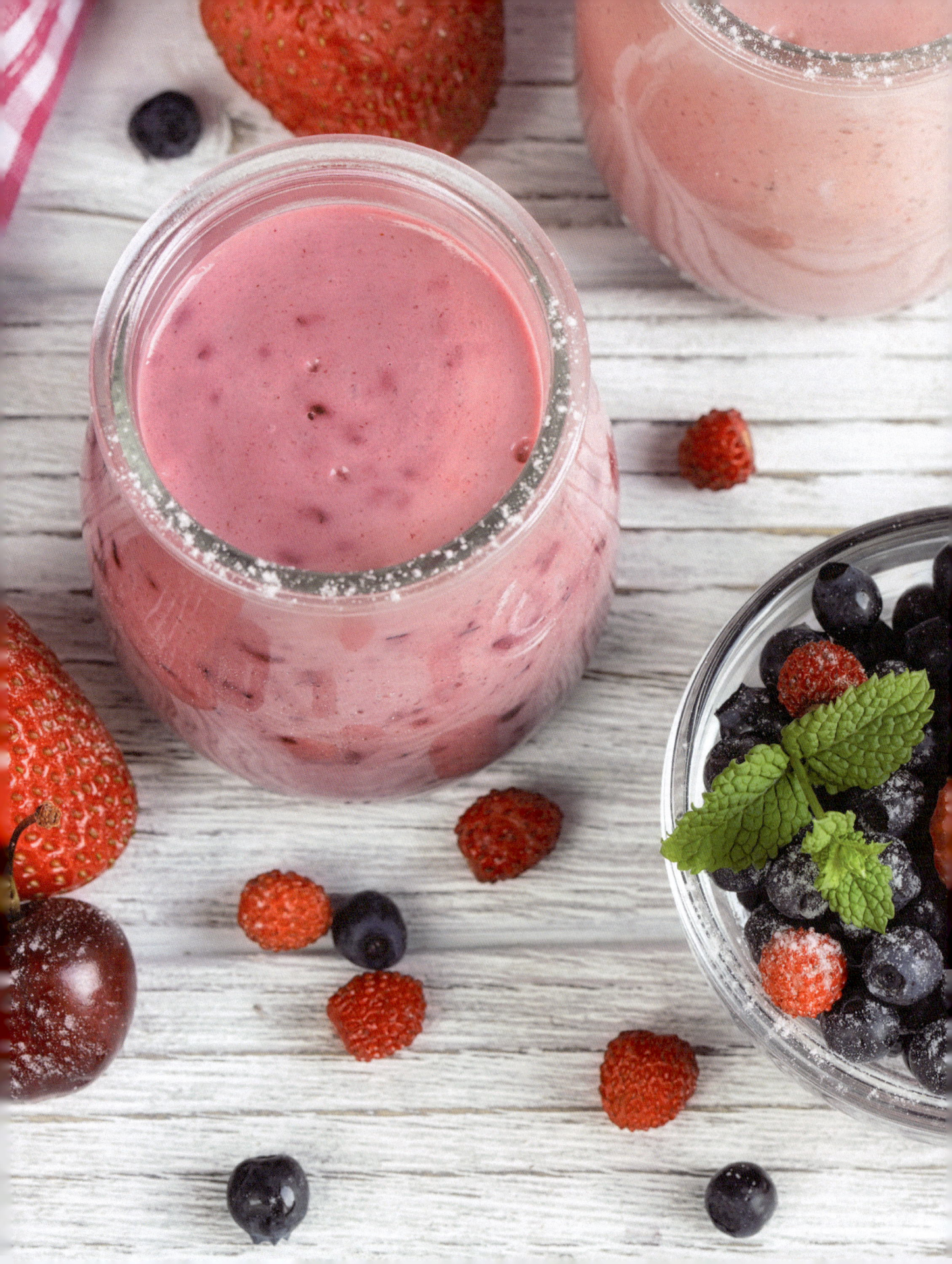

BERRY BOOST SMOOTHIE   Serves 1

INGREDIENTS:

1 cup coconut milk

1/2 cup coconut yoghurt

1/2 cup blueberries

1/2 cup blackberries

1/2 cup strawberries

1/2 cup raspberries

1 scoop of rice protein powder

2 tbsp honey

Salt (to taste)

METHOD:

- Combine all ingredients in a blender. Add more milk if the consistency is too thick.
- Serve immediately.
- If the shake is too bitter, try blending in a bit of salt and honey.
- Also try adding some organic collagen powder for an additional protein boost and thicker consistency.

CLEARLY CITRUS JUICE

Serves 1

INGREDIENTS:

3 oranges, peeled
2 blood oranges, peeled
2 grapefruits, peeled
1/4 lime, juiced
1/4 lemon, juiced

METHOD:

- Juice all of the ingredients into a glass. Mix before drinking. Serve cold.

- Add some salt or honey for extra sweetness if desired.

> "One cannot think well, love well, sleep well, if one has not dined well."
>
> – VIRGINIA WOOLF

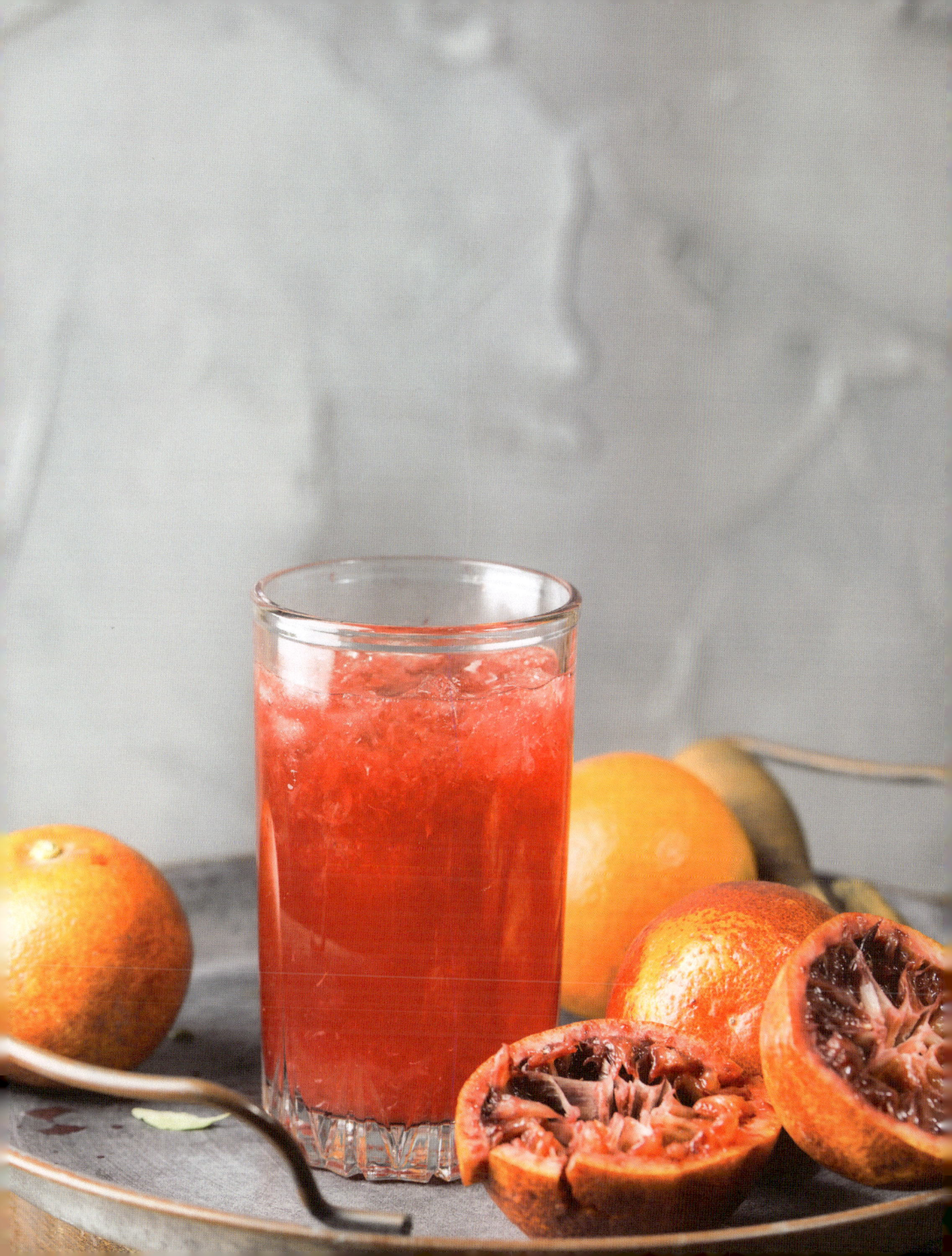

BRITISH FRUIT & VEG SMOOTHIE   Serves 1

INGREDIENTS:

1 cup watercress
3 rhubarb ribs
1 apple, cored
2 pears, cored
2 celery ribs

METHOD:

- Combine the ingredients in a blender for 30 seconds until smooth. Serve cold.
- Add some salt or honey for extra sweetness if desired.

"The only real stumbling block is fear of failure. In cooking you've got to have a what-the-hell attitude."

- JULIA CHILD

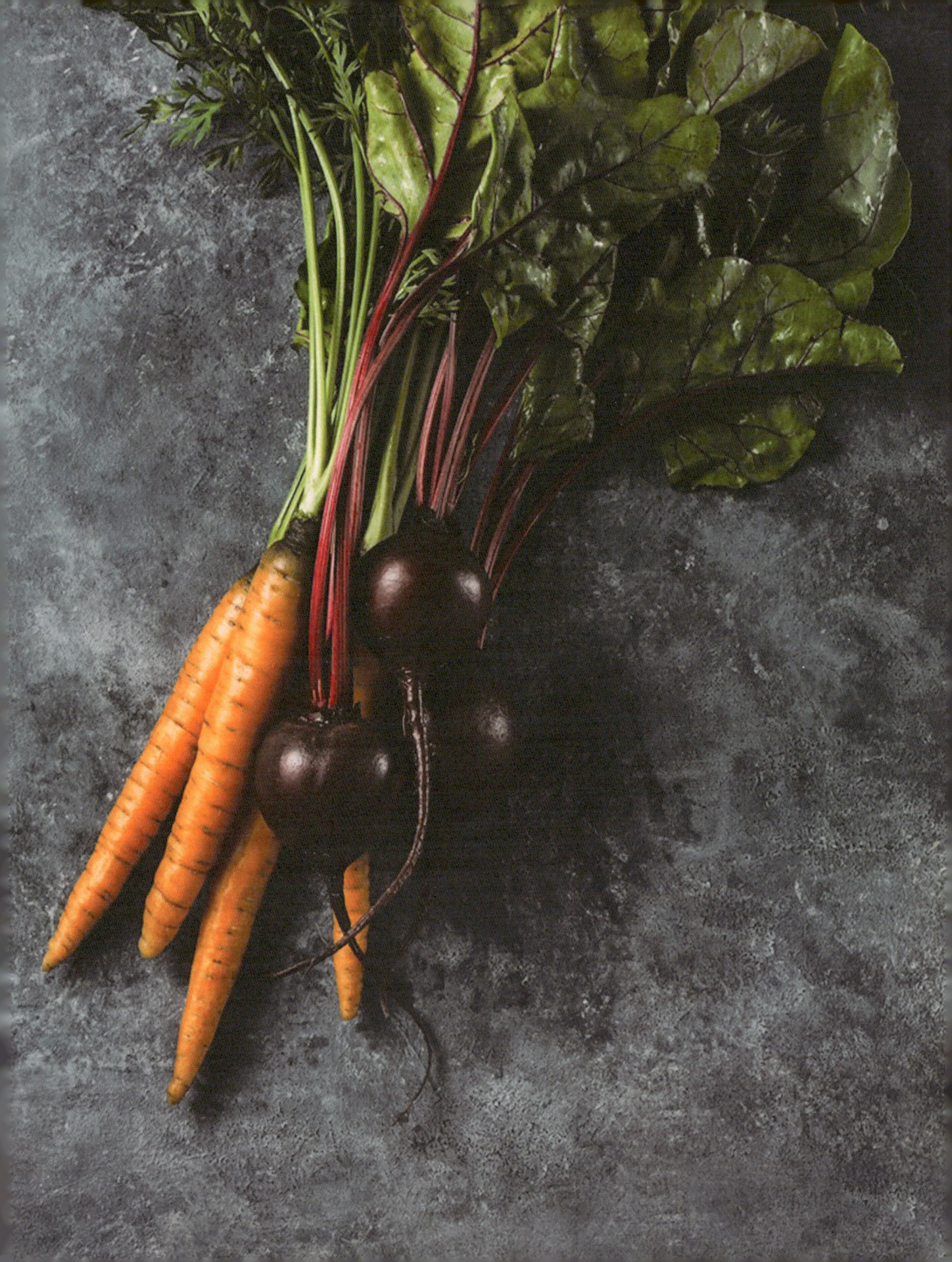

ROYAL ROOT JUICE   Serves 1

INGREDIENTS:

1 tsp ginger, peeled
3 carrots
3 beetroots, peeled
1 apple, cored
1/2 lemon, juiced

METHOD:

- Juice each ingredient into a glass. Make sure it's fully combined. Serve cold.
- Add some salt or honey for extra sweetness if desired.

PINK PUNCH SMOOTHIE — Serves 1

INGREDIENTS:

1 tbsp mint, chopped
3 grapefruits, peeled
8 cherries, pitted
2 pink guavas, peeled
1/2 pineapple, peeled

METHOD:

- Combine the ingredients in a blender for 30 seconds until smooth. Serve cold.
- Add some salt or honey for extra sweetness if desired.

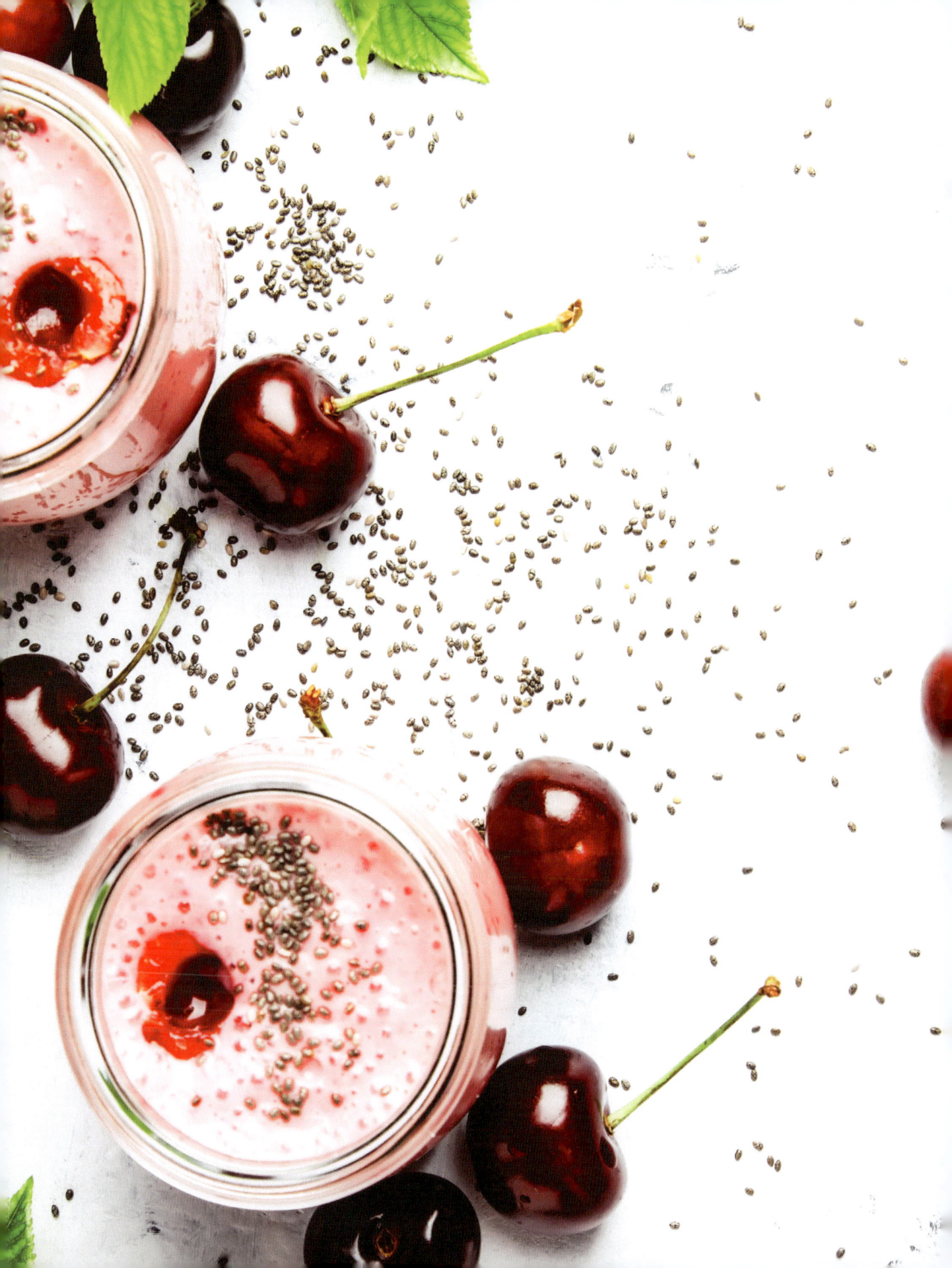

"A balanced diet is a (wheat-free/gluten-free) cookie in each hand."

—BARBARA JOHNSON

TOMATO JUICE Serves 1

INGREDIENTS:

10 medium tomatoes
20 cherry tomatoes
1 tbsp watercress
1 tbsp parsley

METHOD:

- Place all the ingredients into a blender for 30 seconds. Then pour into a tall chilled glass. Make sure it's fully combined. Serve cold.

- Add some salt or honey for extra sweetness if desired.

"At home I serve the kind of food I know the story behind."

– MICHAEL POLLAN

TANGY APPLE JUICE — Serves 1

INGREDIENTS

4 apples, cored
1 tbsp apple cider vinegar
1/2 cup coconut water

METHOD:

- Place all the ingredients into a blender for 30 seconds and pour into a tall chilled glass. Mix with the vinegar and coconut water before drinking. Serve cold.
- Add some salt or honey for extra sweetness if desired.

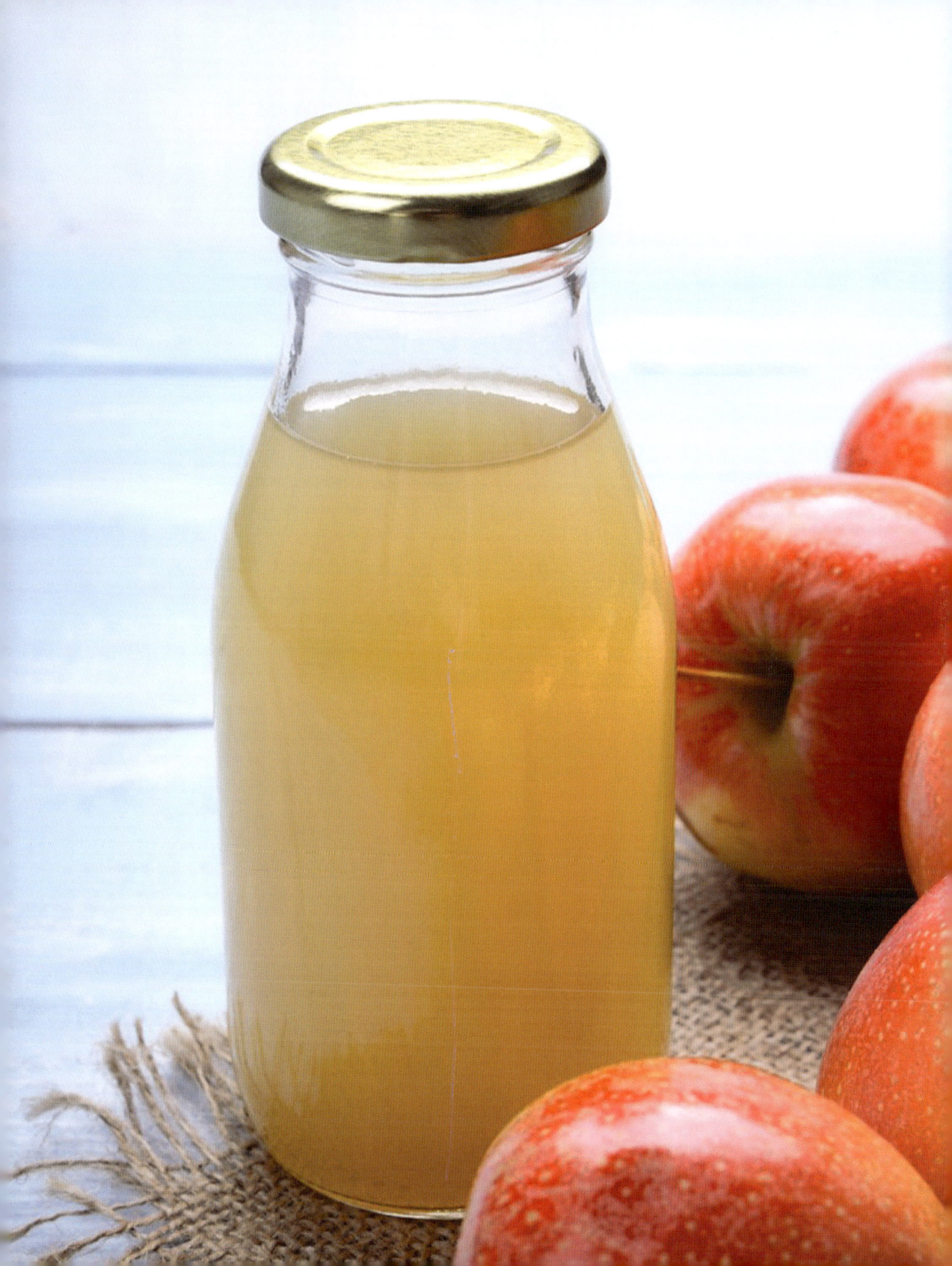

COCONUT & PINEAPPLE SMOOTHIE   Serves 1

INGREDIENTS:

1 cup pineapple, peeled, chopped

1/2 cup thick coconut milk

1 banana, sliced

1/2 cup desiccated coconut

METHOD:

- Mix the ingredients in a blender for 30 seconds. Leave in the refrigerator overnight. Serve cold.
- Add some salt or honey for extra sweetness if desired.

"Tell me what you eat, and I will tell you what you are."

— ANTHELME BRILLAT SAVARIN

'VERY MUCH VEGETABLES' JUICE   Serves 1

INGREDIENTS

2 tomatoes

3 carrots

1 cucumber

1 red pepper, pitted

1 cup spinach

1 cup kale

4 celery ribs

METHOD:

- Place all the ingredients into a blender for 30 seconds and pour into a tall chilled glass. Mix before drinking. Serve cold.
- Add some salt or honey for extra sweetness if desired.

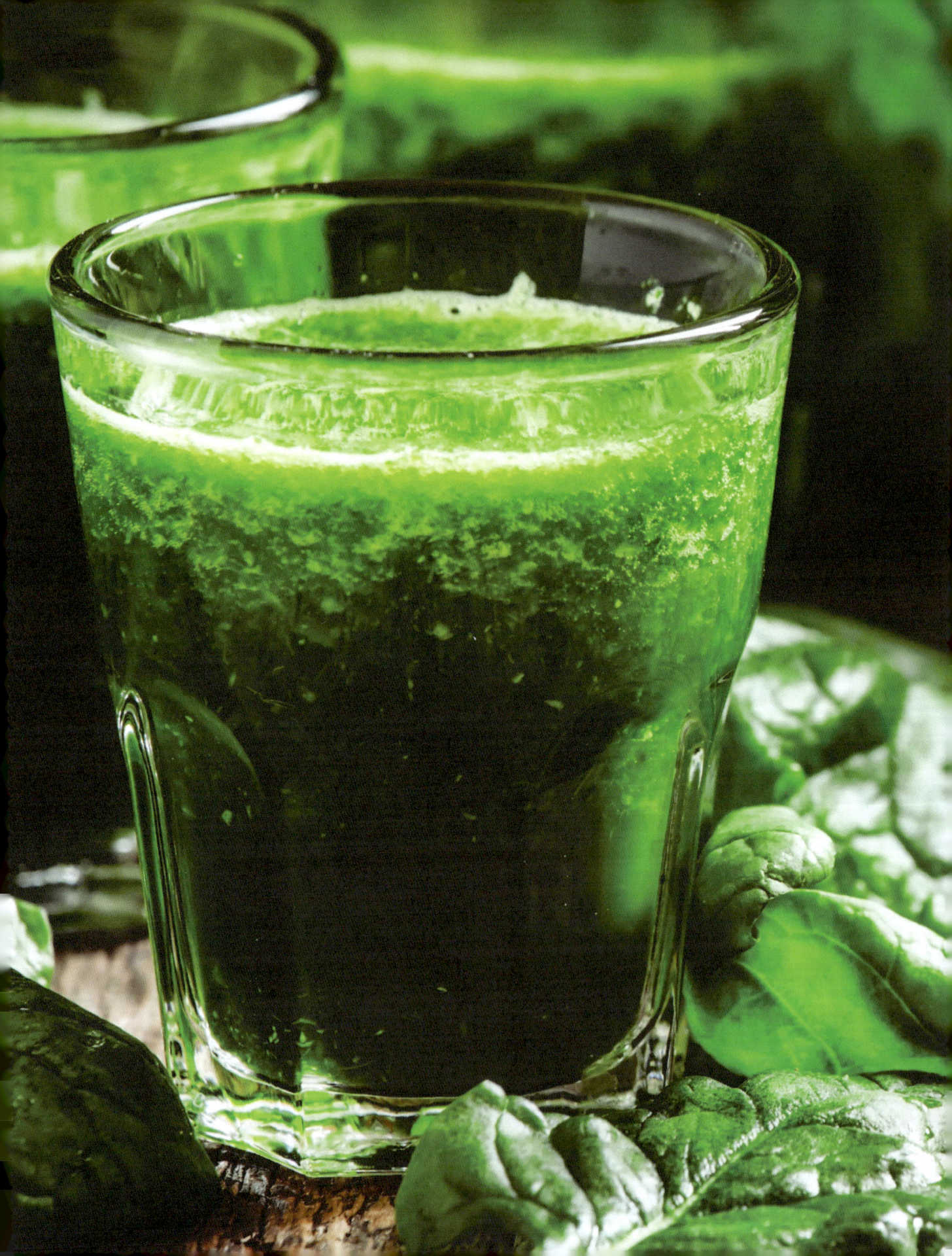

LUSCIOUS LEAFY GREEN JUICE   Serves 1

INGREDIENTS

3 cups spinach

2 cups romaine lettuce

2 cups coconut water

3 cups kale

METHOD:

- Place all the ingredients into a blender for 30 seconds and pour into a tall chilled glass. Mix before drinking. Serve cold.

- Add some salt or honey for extra sweetness if desired.

SUPER SONIC GREEN SHAKE — Serves 1

INGREDIENTS:

2 cups spinach
1 celery stalk, chopped
1 cup green grapes
1 green apple, chopped
1 cucumber, chopped

1 cup milk

METHOD:

- Combine all ingredients in a blender. Add more milk if the consistency is too thick. Serve immediately.
- If the shake is too bitter, try blending in a bit of salt and honey.

Mix with some protein powder for a protein boost or enjoy alongside the pancakes recipe.

"Food should be fun."

– THOMAS KELLER

'RED VELVET' SHAKE   Serves 1

INGREDIENTS:

2 cups spinach

2 carrots, diced

1 large tomato

1 cup strawberries

1 cup raspberries

1 beetroot, peeled, diced

1 cup milk

METHOD:

- Combine all ingredients in a blender. Add more milk if the consistency is too thick. Serve immediately.
- If the shake is too bitter, try blending in a bit of salt and honey.

Mix with some protein powder for a protein boost or enjoy alongside the pancakes recipe.

STRAWBERRY PROTEIN SMOOTHIE   Serves 1

INGREDIENTS

1 cup of strawberries
2 cups coconut milk
1 scoop rice protein powder
1 tbsp honey

METHOD:

- Put all the ingredients in a blender and mix for 30 seconds.
- Loosen with more coconut water or milk if necessary.
- Add some salt or honey for extra sweetness if desired.

"As for butter versus margarine; I trust cows more than chemists."

– JOAN GUSSOW

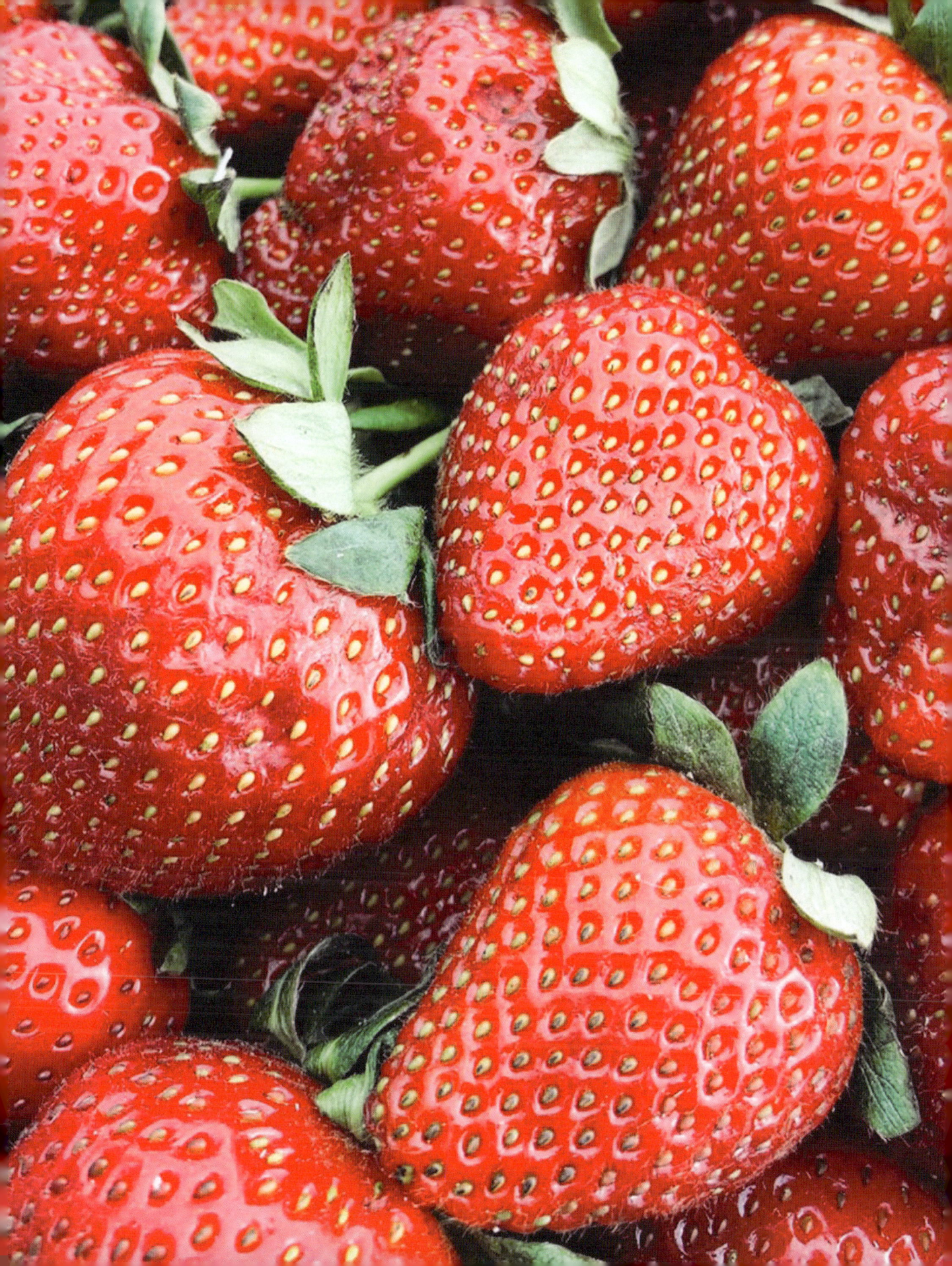

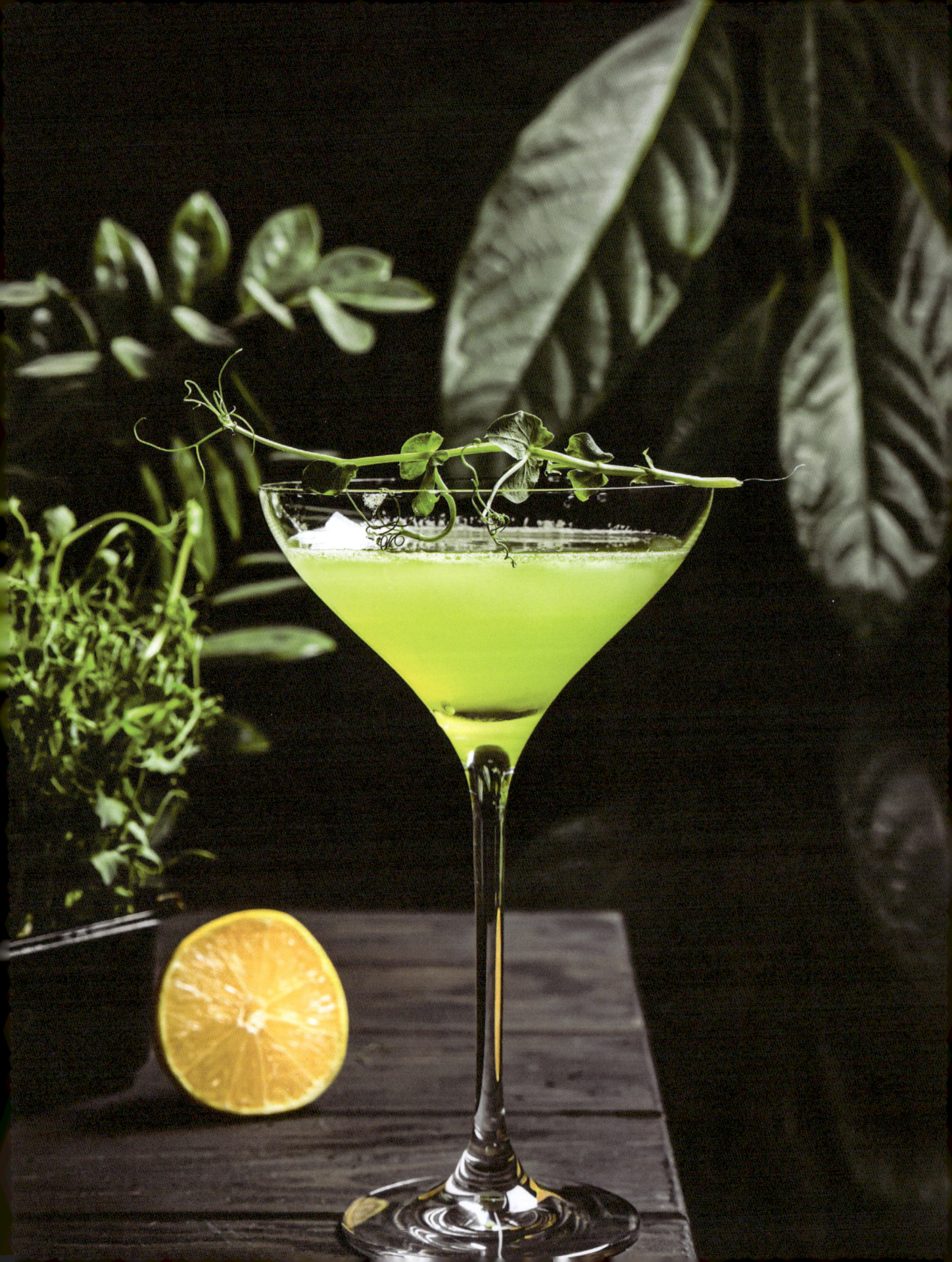

MARVELOUS MEXICAN MOCKTAIL

Inspired by **EndoBoss® Alumni & Coach** - Marie West from UK   Serves 1

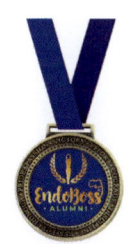

INGREDIENTS:

1 cup spinach
1/4 cucumber, sliced
2 celery ribs, diced
1 apple, cored
1/2 orange (or lime), juiced

1 tbsp mint, chopped

METHOD:

- Combine all the ingredients in a blender for a few minutes until smooth.
- You may wish to add 1 cup full of blended ice for an authentic cocktail feel.
- Add some salt or honey for extra sweetness if desired.

"When eating fruit, remember who planted the tree."

– VIETNAMESE PROVERB

HYDRATION STATION SHAKE — Serves 1

INGREDIENTS:

1 cucumber, diced
1/4 cup coconut water
1/2 watermelon, skinned
Salt (to taste)

METHOD:

- Combine all ingredients in a blender. Add more milk if the consistency is too thick. Serve immediately.
- If the shake is too bitter, try blending in a bit of salt and honey.

Mix with some protein powder for a protein boost or enjoy alongside the pancakes recipe.

LUSCIOUS LUNCHES & SALADS

"The act of putting into your mouth what the earth has grown is perhaps your most direct interaction with earth."

– FRANCES MOORE LAPPE

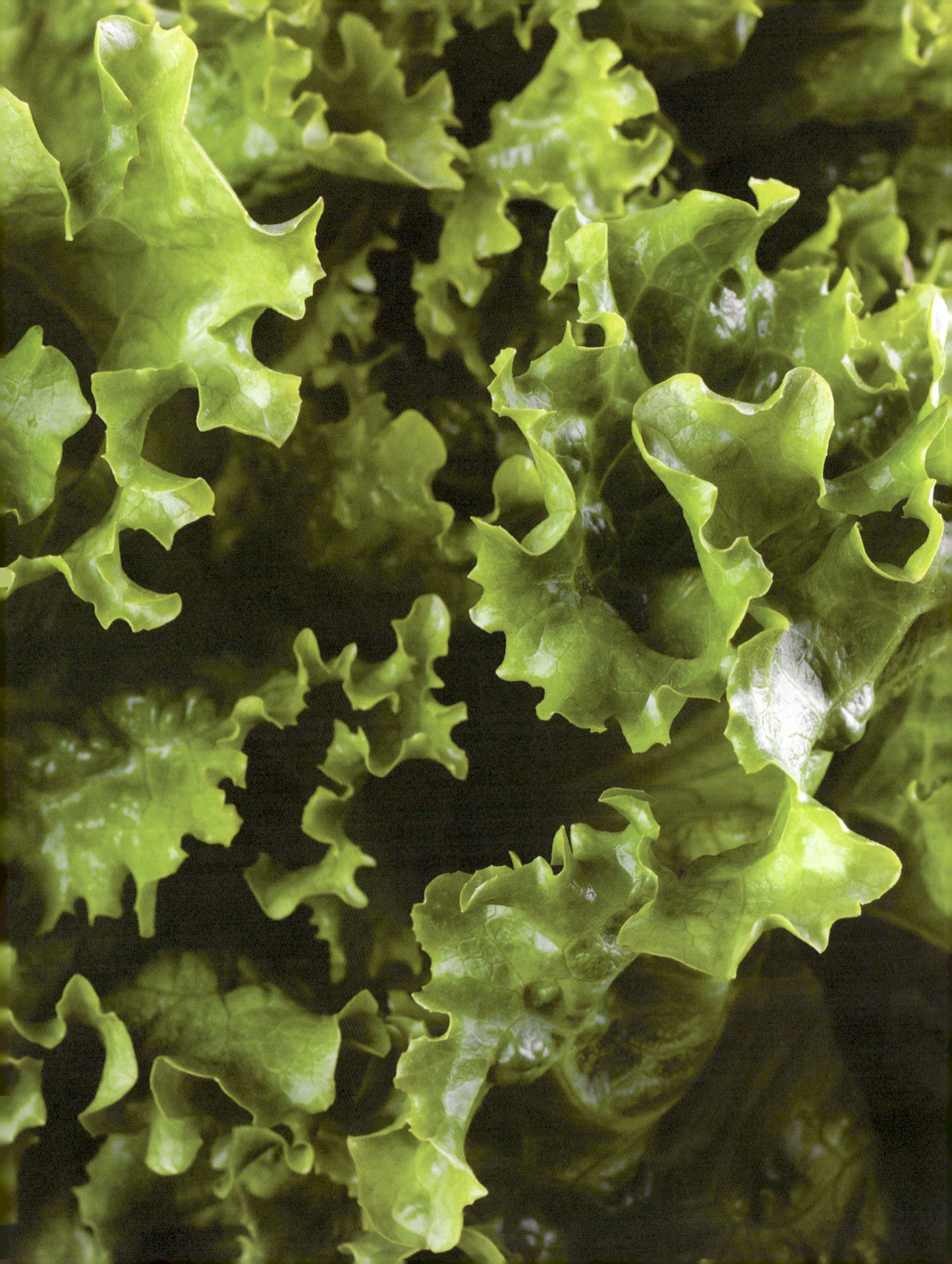

GREEN TUNA SALAD   Serves 2

INGREDIENTS:

1 tin of tuna
1/2 celery rib, diced
1 tbsp red onion, diced
2 tbsp chives
3 cups spinach

1 tbsp honey
1/2 tbsp Dijon mustard
1 avocado, mashed
1/2 cup green beans
Salt (to taste)

METHOD:

- Bring a pot of water to the boil. Salt the water and then add the beans. Cook until tender. This should take about 5 minutes. Remove from the heat and drain.

- Meanwhile, in a small bowl, combine the avocado, mustard, honey and some salt. Then spoon in the tuna, red onion, chives and celery, and mix again.

- Get a large plate or bowl and add the spinach and green beans onto it. Spoon over the tuna mix and enjoy!

TOMATO & MOZZARELLA SALAD — Serves 2

INGREDIENTS:

1 chicken breast
1 ball of mozzarella, torn
1/4 cup red onion, diced
1 bell pepper, cored, seeded, diced
1 tbsp lemon juice
1 1/2 cups tomatoes, diced
2 tbsp capers

1 tbsp extra virgin olive oil
1 celery rib, diced
1 cup mixed lettuce
1 cup rocket
1 tbsp coconut oil
Balsamic vinegar (to taste)
Salt (to taste)

METHOD:

- Preheat the oven to 200°C. Salt the chicken breast and place in an ovenproof dish with the coconut oil. Cook in the oven until cooked through. Spoon the oil over the chicken every ten minutes to keep it moist.

- Meanwhile, in a small bowl, combine the bell pepper, tomatoes, celery, capers, onion, olive oil and lemon juice.

- Get a large plate or bowl and add the rocket and lettuce. Spoon over the tomato and caper mix. Tear the mozzarella and place on top.

- When the chicken is done, slice the chicken into strips and add on top of the salad. Drizzle the salad with some balsamic vinegar. Enjoy!

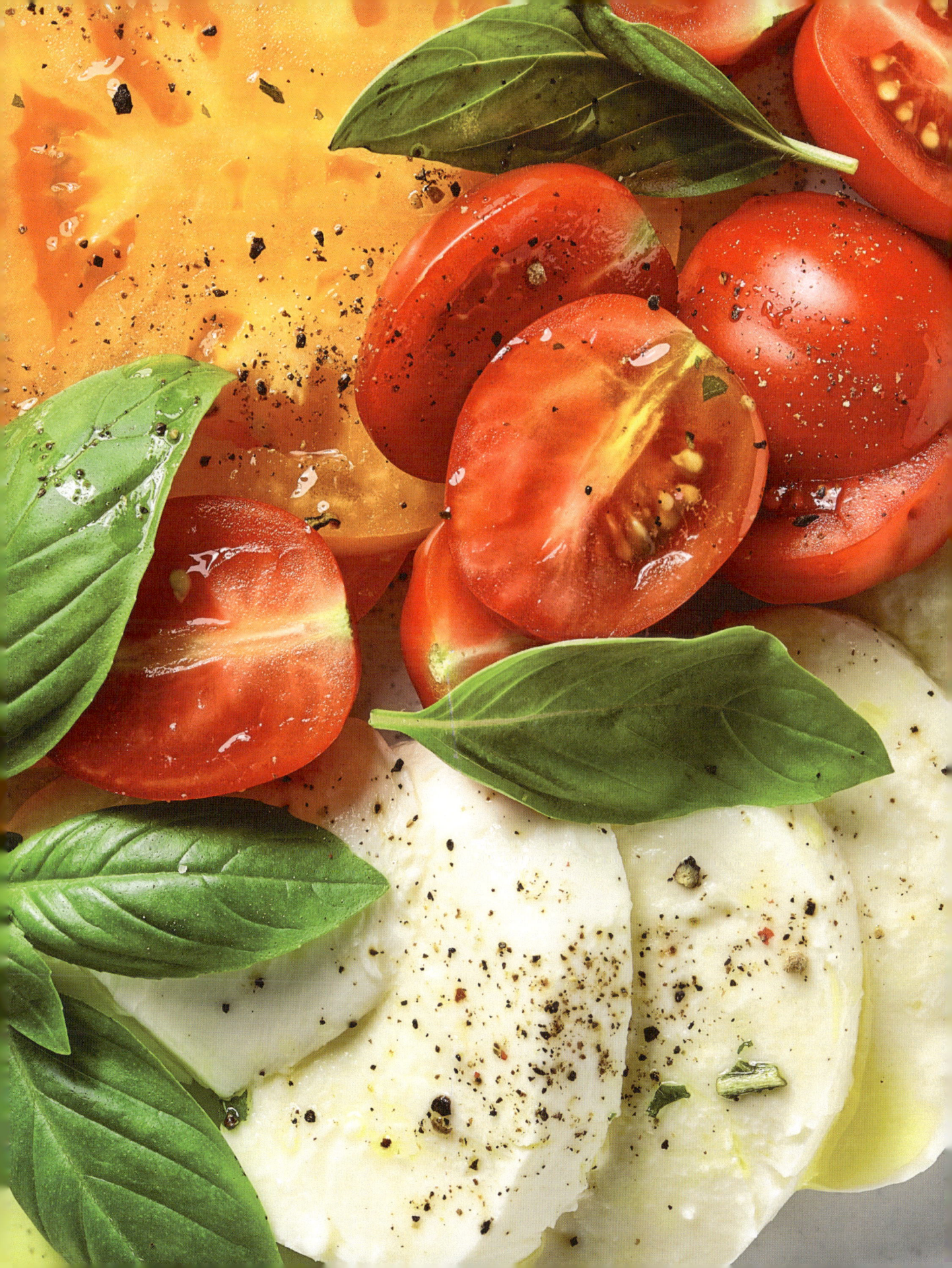

SWEET AND CRUNCHY BEEF SALAD   Serves 2

INGREDIENTS:

7oz beef steak
1 tbsp lime juice
1/2 tsp lime zest
1 tsp honey
1 small red onion, thinly sliced
8 sprigs coriander, chopped
10 cherry tomatoes, quartered
1/3 cup thick coconut milk

1/2 mango, peeled, cubed
1 spring onion, thinly sliced
1 apple
1 tbsp coconut oil
3 tbsp desiccated coconut
1 cup mixed lettuce
Salt (to taste)

METHOD:

- Rinse the sliced onion under some water and mix in a bowl with the lime juice, lime zest, and honey. Set aside in the fridge.

- Heat a frying pan over a medium to high heat, add in the coconut oil and then fry the steak. I recommend cooking the steak to rare which takes about 2 minutes each side. Once done, remove from the heat and set aside.

- Add the mango, coconut milk, spring onion and coriander to the onion mixture. Set aside in the fridge again.

- Meanwhile, chop the apple into thin matchsticks and then mix with the desiccated coconut.

- On a plate, lay out the lettuce, top with the mango and onion mixture, and then add the coconut apple mix and the tomatoes. Finally, slice the steak and lay on top.

PORK CHOPS & SWEET POTATO DISH

Inspired by **EndoBoss® Alumni** - Laura Majugo Muhwezi from Uganda

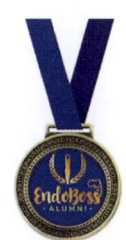

Serves 2

INGREDIENTS:

4 pork chops

2 carrots, diced

3 tbsp coconut oil

2 large tomatoes, quartered

2 red onions, diced

2 large sweet potatoes, diced

5 garlic cloves

Pepper (to taste)

Salt (to taste)

METHOD:

- Salt the pork chops. Preheat the oven to 180°C.

- Grind the tomatoes and garlic together into a smooth paste.

- Next, get a large bowl and mix the tomato paste, carrots, onions, potatoes, and coconut oil. Add in the pork chops. Add salt and pepper to taste. Allow the mix to sit for around 30 minutes before transferring to an oven tray.

- Cook for around 45 minutes until the pork is cooked through and slightly golden. Serve hot.

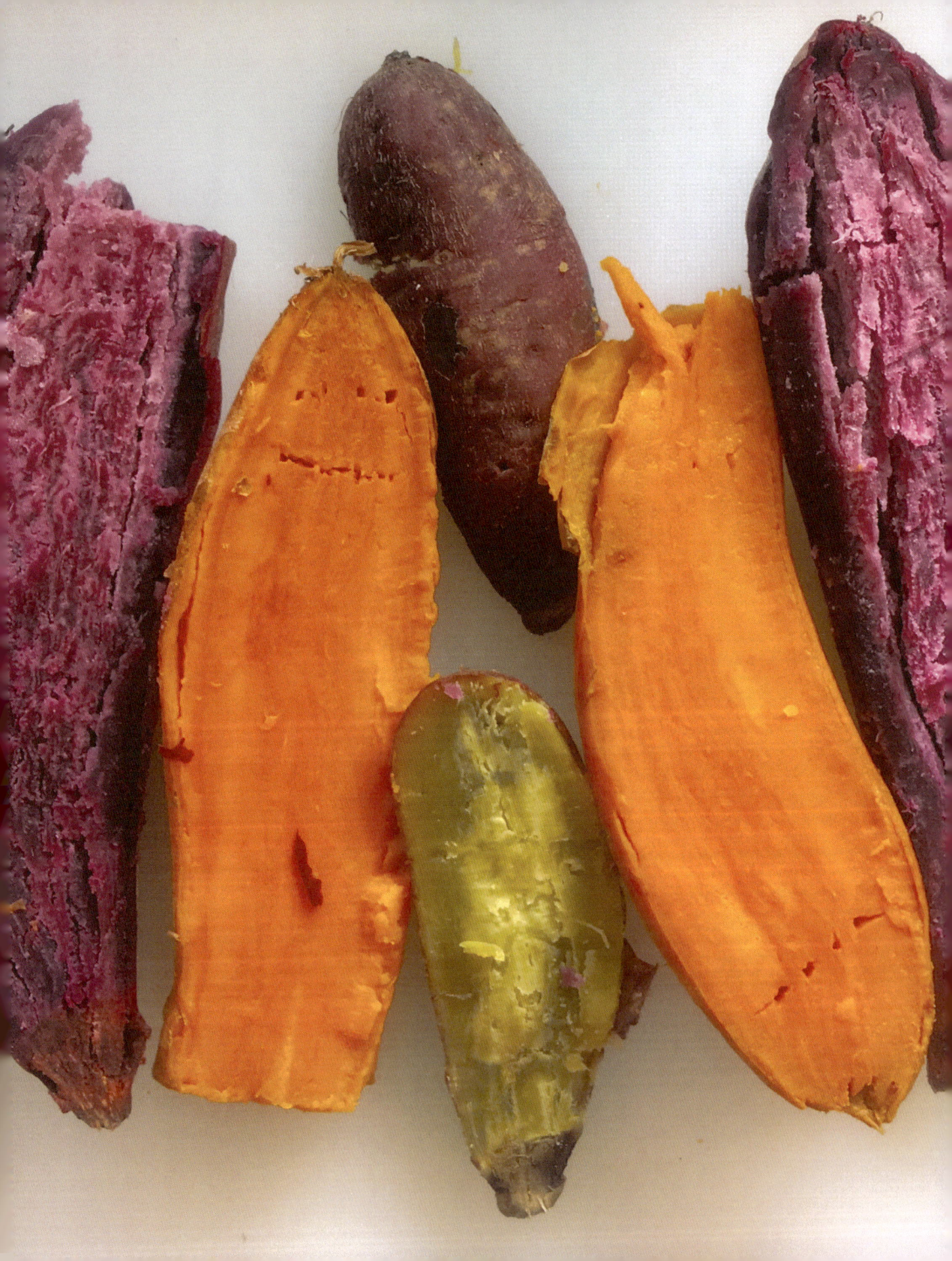

"When baking, follow directions. When cooking, go by your own taste."

– LAIKO BAHRS

CHICKEN & LEEK PIES

Inspired by **EndoBoss® Alumni** - Nadja Ilic from Germany

Serves 4-6

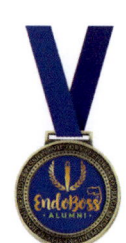

INGREDIENTS:

- 2 chicken thighs
- 2 cups potato flour
- 1/2 cup water
- 2 tsp baking powder
- 2 tsp gelatin powder
- 2 tbsp coconut oil
- 1 onion, diced
- 1 garlic clove, minced
- 2 leeks, halved, sliced
- 2 cups rice flour
- 1 tsp Dijon mustard
- 1/4 cup cheese, grated
- 3/4 cup olive oil
- 1 egg, beaten
- Pepper (to taste)
- Salt (to taste)

METHOD:

- Salt the chicken. Preheat the oven to 180°C. To make the pastry, add the flour, baking powder, gelatin and some salt to a bowl.

- Gradually mix in the olive oil and then the water 1 tbsp at a time. Knead well until the dough is smooth. Stop adding water if the dough becomes too soft. Cover and rest in the fridge.

- Next, prepare the filling. Place the chicken on an oven tray with 1 tbsp coconut oil and cook in the oven for around 20 minutes until just cooked through. Then, shred with two forks and set aside.

- Meanwhile, heat a frying pan with the remaining coconut oil and add the leeks, onion, garlic and some salt and pepper. Cook until all the vegetables have softened or are aromatic.

- Mix the cooked vegetables and chicken in a bowl with the cheese and mustard. Combine well and add more salt and pepper if desired.

- Make the dough into six equally sized balls and press them into individual rectangles. Spoon in the filling to each. Pinch the sides and fold over the dough to create individual pies. Pierce each in a few spots and then brush with the beaten egg. Bake in the oven for around 40 minutes until the dough is golden.

CHEESY CHICKEN NACHOS WITH GUACAMOLE & SALSA   Serves 4

INGREDIENTS:

3 cooked chicken thighs, shredded
6 spring onions, thinly sliced
2 tbsp corianders, chopped
1 lime, juiced
2 avocados, skinned, pitted
6 large tomatoes, finely chopped
1 red onion, finely diced
1 garlic clove, minced

1 tsp white wine vinegar
1 1/2 cups cheddar cheese, grated
1 1/4 cups rice tortilla chips (preferably fried in coconut oil or tallow not vegetable/seed oil!)
Pepper (to taste)
Salt (to taste)

METHOD:

- Preheat the oven to 180°C. In an ovenproof dish, layer the tortilla chips with the cheese, cooked chicken thighs and spring onions. Place in the oven for 5-10 minutes, until the cheese has melted.

- Meanwhile, to make the guacamole, combine the avocado, half the lime juice, 1 chopped tomato, 1 tbsp coriander, half the diced red onion and some salt and pepper in a bowl. Mix well until a smooth paste forms.

- Next, for the salsa, add the other tomatoes, garlic, remaining lime juice, vinegar, remaining onion and 1 tbsp coriander to a bowl and combine well.

- Once the nachos are done, serve immediately with the guacamole and salsa.

SMOKED MACKEREL NIÇOISE SALAD   Serves 2

INGREDIENTS:

2 smoked mackerel fillets
2 cups baby potatoes, halved
2/3 cup green beans, trimmed
3 eggs
2/3 cup cherry tomatoes, halved
1/4 cup black olives, pitted, halved
1 tsp dijon mustard

1 garlic clove
1/2 lemon, juiced
3 cups mixed salad
5 tbsp olive oil
Pepper (to taste)
Salt (to taste)

METHOD:

- Preheat the oven to 200°C.
- Place the potatoes in the oven with 1 tbsp of olive oil, and salt and pepper. Cook until soft and golden.
- Next, bring a pot of salted water to the boil. Add in the green beans and cook until slightly softened (around 3 minutes). Once done, remove from the pan and add in the eggs.
- Boil for the desired yolk consistency (around 5 minutes for soft and 9 minutes for hard). Plunge in cold water once cooked, and then quarter.
- To make the dressing, mix the lemon juice, garlic, mustard, 4 tbsp olive oil, and some salt and pepper together.
- Assemble the dish by plating the salad leaves, then artfully arrange the potatoes, olives, tomatoes, green beans, eggs and mackerel on the plate. Finally, drizzle with the dressing (to taste).

CRISPY PANCETTA & FETA STUFFED PEPPERS   Serves 2

INGREDIENTS:

- 1/2 cup feta goats cheese, crumbled
- 1 tbsp coconut oil
- 1/2 red onion, diced
- 1 garlic clove, minced
- 1/2 tomato, chopped
- 1 tbsp chopped parsley
- 1 tbsp olive oil
- 2/3 cup pancetta, diced
- 2 large bell peppers

METHOD:

- Preheat the oven to 180°C. Heat a small frying pan over a medium heat and cook the pancetta until it starts to crisp. Once ready, remove from the heat and set the pancetta aside. Reserve the fat from the pan.

- To make the stuffing, mix the pancetta, olive oil, onion, garlic, feta, parsley and tomato in a large bowl.

- Slice across the top of the peppers to create an entrance for the stuffing, like a lid. Remove the seeds, core and pith (white parts). Spoon in the stuffing.

- Brush the peppers with the reserved pancetta fat and put the tops back on the peppers. Place in an ovenproof dish that has been smeared with the coconut oil.

- Cook for about 25-30 minutes or until the pepper is soft and nicely coloured, and the cheese has melted.

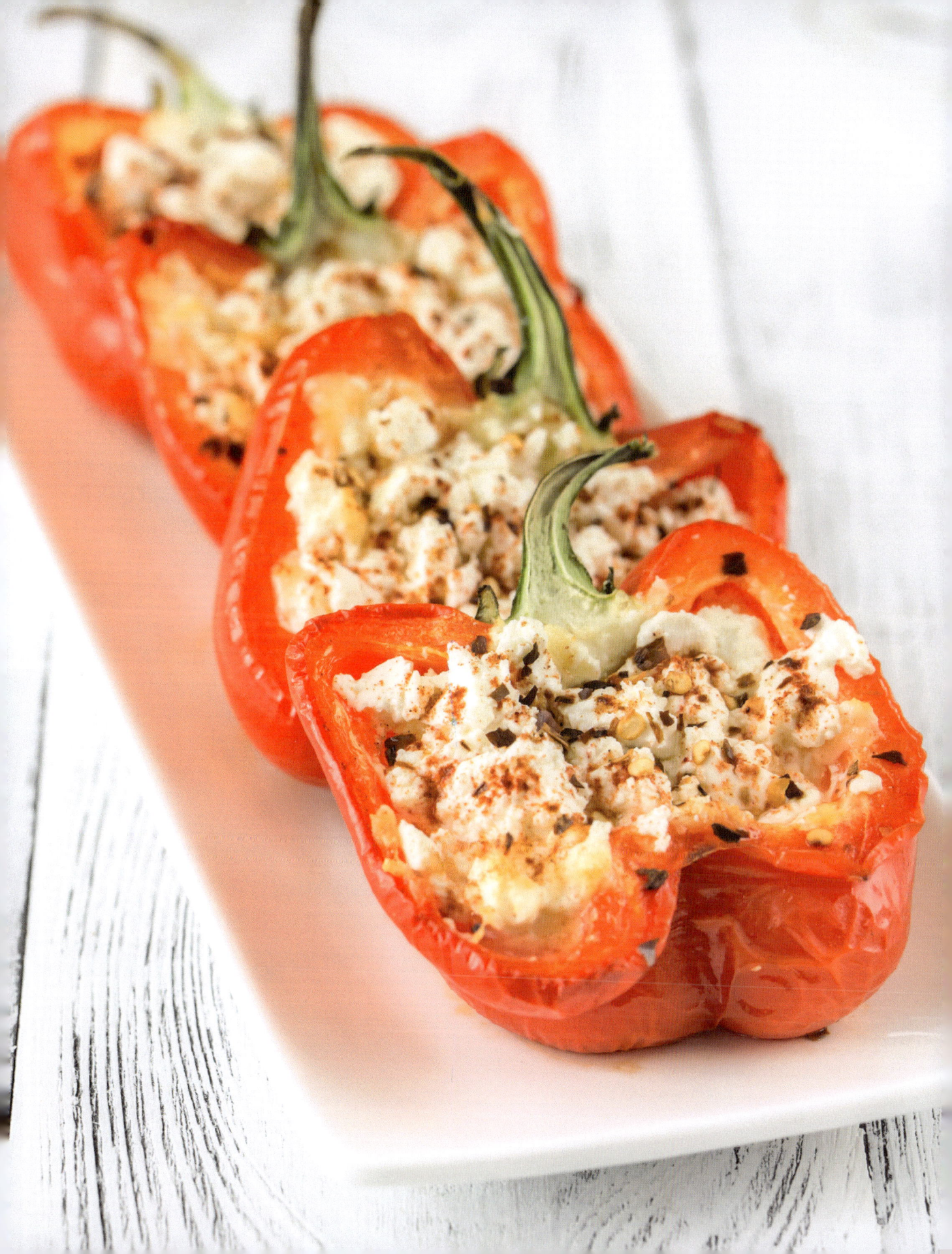

TURKEY SQUASH SALAD — Serves 4

INGREDIENTS:

- 1 butternut squash, peeled, seeded
- 1 tbsp paprika
- 2 1/2 cups roasted turkey meat
- 5 cups rocket
- 2 avocados, peeled, cubed
- 1 cup sun-dried tomatoes, halved
- 2/3 cup hard cheese, grated
- 1/2 cup black olives, pitted, halved
- 2 tbsp apple cider vinegar
- 2 tbsp honey
- 1 tbsp coconut oil
- 1 tbsp extra virgin olive oil
- Pepper (to taste)
- Salt (to taste)

METHOD:

- Preheat the oven to 200°C. Chop the butternut squash into 2 cm cubes and then transfer to an ovenproof dish with some salt, pepper, the coconut oil and paprika. Toast for 30 minutes or until fully soft and slightly golden. When done, allow the squash to cool.

- Meanwhile, make the dressing by combining the olive oil, honey, vinegar and some salt in a small bowl.

- If not already done so, cut the turkey meat into small chunks or thin slices. Begin serving the salad by plating the rocket first, and then topping with the olives, avocado, squash and sun-dried tomatoes. Next, drizzle over the dressing and finally top that with the turkey and cheese.

TOMATO & MUSHROOM BAKE   Serves 2-4

INGREDIENTS:

6 eggs

6 medium tomatoes, quartered

2 cups mushrooms, sliced

2 tbsp coconut oil

1 cup chorizo sausage, chopped

2 garlic cloves, minced

2 tbsp chives, chopped

Pepper (to taste)

Salt (to taste)

METHOD:

- Preheat the oven to 180°C. Grease an oven tray with the coconut oil and then add in the tomatoes, garlic and mushrooms.

- Mix around and then sprinkle with salt and pepper.

- Bake in the oven for around 30 minutes until the vegetables are cooked and soft.

- Once ready, layer on the chorizo before cracking the eggs on top of the entire bake. Take care not to break the yolks.

- Return to the oven for around 5-10 minutes until the egg whites are cooked. Remove from the oven and sprinkle with the chives.

- Serve hot.

TUNACADO BOWL — Serves 2

INGREDIENTS:

- 2 tins of tuna, drained
- 1 avocado, peeled, pitted
- 2 large sweet potatoes, peeled, cubed
- 1 tbsp olive oil
- 2 tbsp coriander, chopped
- 1/2 cucumber, sliced
- Pepper (to taste)
- Salt (to taste)

METHOD:

- Place the sweet potatoes in a pot of salted water and bring to the boil.
- Continue to cook for 10-15 minutes until the potatoes have softened.
- Once done, mash thoroughly. Add pepper and more salt if desired.
- Meanwhile, mash the avocado and mix with the tuna, coriander, olive oil, and some salt and pepper.
- Plate the tunacado in a bowl alongside the mashed sweet potato, and sliced cucumber.

"Learn how to cook – try new recipes, learn from your mistakes, be fearless, and above all have fun!"

– JULIA CHILD

CRUSTLESS QUICHE   Serves 8

INGREDIENTS:

6 eggs
1 small red onion, diced
1 cup shredded cheese
3 cups spinach
1 cup double cream

1 small onion, chopped
2/3 cup of bacon, diced
Pepper (to taste)
Salt (to taste)

METHOD:

- Preheat the oven to 180°C. Grease a pie dish with butter or coconut oil.

- Combine the eggs, cream, salt and pepper. Then add the bacon, spinach, cheese and onion. Mix again and transfer to the pie dish.

- Cook the quiche for between 30-40 minutes or until golden on top. Be careful not to overcook as the quiche will dry out and lose creaminess.

- Remove from the oven and rest for 10 minutes. Cut your desired amount, then serve with green leaf salad and enjoy.

SHEPARD'S PIE   Serves 4-6

INGREDIENTS:

4 cups beef mince
2 tbsp coconut oil
2 carrots, diced
1 bay leaf
1 tbsp tomato puree
1 tbsp rice flour
1/2 cup milk
3 tbsp Worcestershire sauce
7 cups potato, peeled, diced
1 celery ribs, diced
2 garlic cloves, minced
1 onion, diced
1 tbsp butter
1 1/2 cups beef stock
1 cup frozen peas
2/3 cup cheese, grated
Pepper (to taste)
Salt (to taste)

METHOD:

- Salt the beef mince. Preheat the oven to 200°C. Heat 1 tbsp coconut oil in a large frying pan. Tip in the beef and fry until browned. Set aside. Add in the remaining coconut oil to the pan and cook the onions, carrots, and celery with some salt and pepper, for about 15 minutes. Add the garlic and cook for a further 5 minutes.

- Next, return the beef to the pan along with the flour, tomato puree, stock, Worcestershire sauce and bay leaf. Bring to the boil and then simmer, uncovered, for 30 minutes until a thick gravy forms. Once done, discard the bay leaf. Adjust the seasoning if necessary.

- Meanwhile, place the potatoes in a pot of salted water and bring to the boil. Simmer for about 10-15 minutes until tender. Drain and then mash with the milk, butter and 1/2 cup of the cheese. Season again if necessary.

- Spoon the mince into an ovenproof dish (or into many small ones for convenient single servings) and then dollop the mash on top to cover the mince. Sprinkle with the remaining cheese. Place in the oven for about 20-30 minutes until the mash is crisp and golden on top. Serve hot. Enjoy!

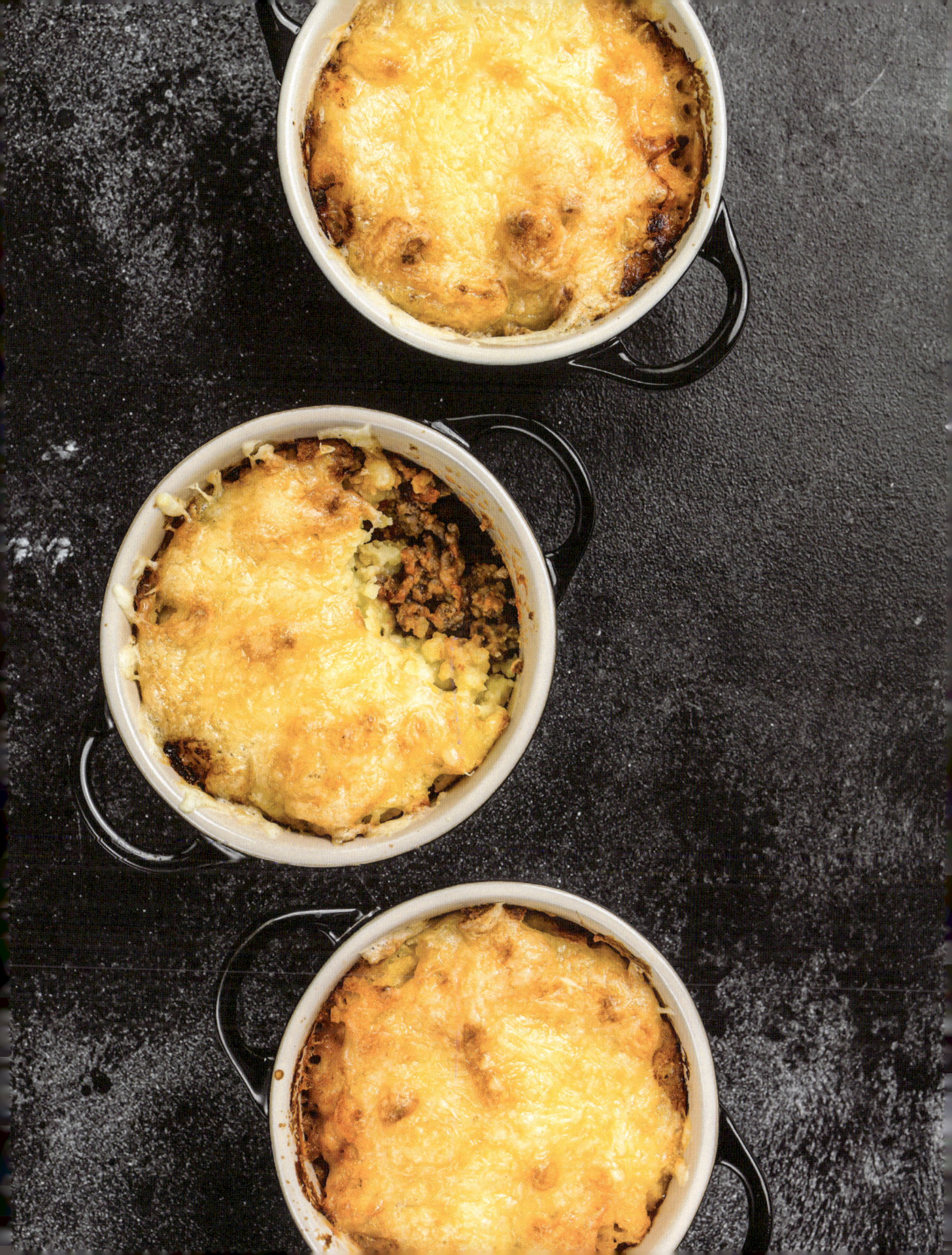

SUPER BURGERS & WEDGES   Serves 2

INGREDIENTS:

- 2 beef burger patties
- Head of iceberg lettuce
- 1 small red onion, sliced
- 2 eggs
- 4 large potatoes (around 6 cups)
- 2 tbsp coconut oil
- 1 1/2 tbsp balsamic vinegar
- 2 tbsp honey
- 1 large tomato, sliced
- 4 slices of cheese (or 2/3 cup sliced)
- 1 gherkin, sliced
- Ketchup (to taste)
- Mustard (to taste)
- Salt (to taste)

METHOD:

- Preheat the oven to 200°C. Place the burgers on a grill in an oven tray and cook for 25 minutes.

- Slice the potatoes into wedges. Place on an oven tray with some salt and half the coconut oil. Cook until golden and the outside is crisp.

- Heat up a small frying pan with a quarter of the coconut oil and some salt. Add the red onion and fry until softened, then add the honey and the balsamic vinegar. Cook until the honey and balsamic reduces into a thick liquid. Remove from the pan and set aside. Reheat the pan with the remaining coconut oil and fry the eggs. Set aside when done.

- Get the lettuce and remove a few of the outer layers. Next, chop about 1/2 inch off the base of the lettuce. Peel off the leaves whilst making sure to keep them intact.

- To assemble the burgers, lay some lettuce on a plate and place a beef patty on top. Add on two slices of cheese, then the sliced tomato, the balsamic red onions, and finally a fried egg. Add some mustard, ketchup and gherkins to your personal liking, and then cover with more lettuce.

"If organic farming is the natural way, shouldn't organic produce just be called 'produce' and make the pesticide-laden stuff take the burden of an adjective?"

– YMBER DELECTO

LUNCH ON THE MOVE*

Shop ideas

- Pre-made salad with some cooked chicken
- Sushi
- Tinned tuna in spring water
- Tinned mackerel or sardines
- Pre-boiled eggs
- Dried chicken, beef or pork crisps/chips
- Coconut water or fresh fruit juice

Equally, if there is a small deli near you that uses fresh, quality ingredients you may be able to find some great takeaway options like soups and salads.

*Refer back to our 'breakfast on the move' list for other suggestions or check out our soup section for some great soups that can be enjoyed for lunch.

DELICIOUS DINNERS & MAINS

"The only time to eat diet food is while you're waiting for the steak to cook."

— JULIA CHILD

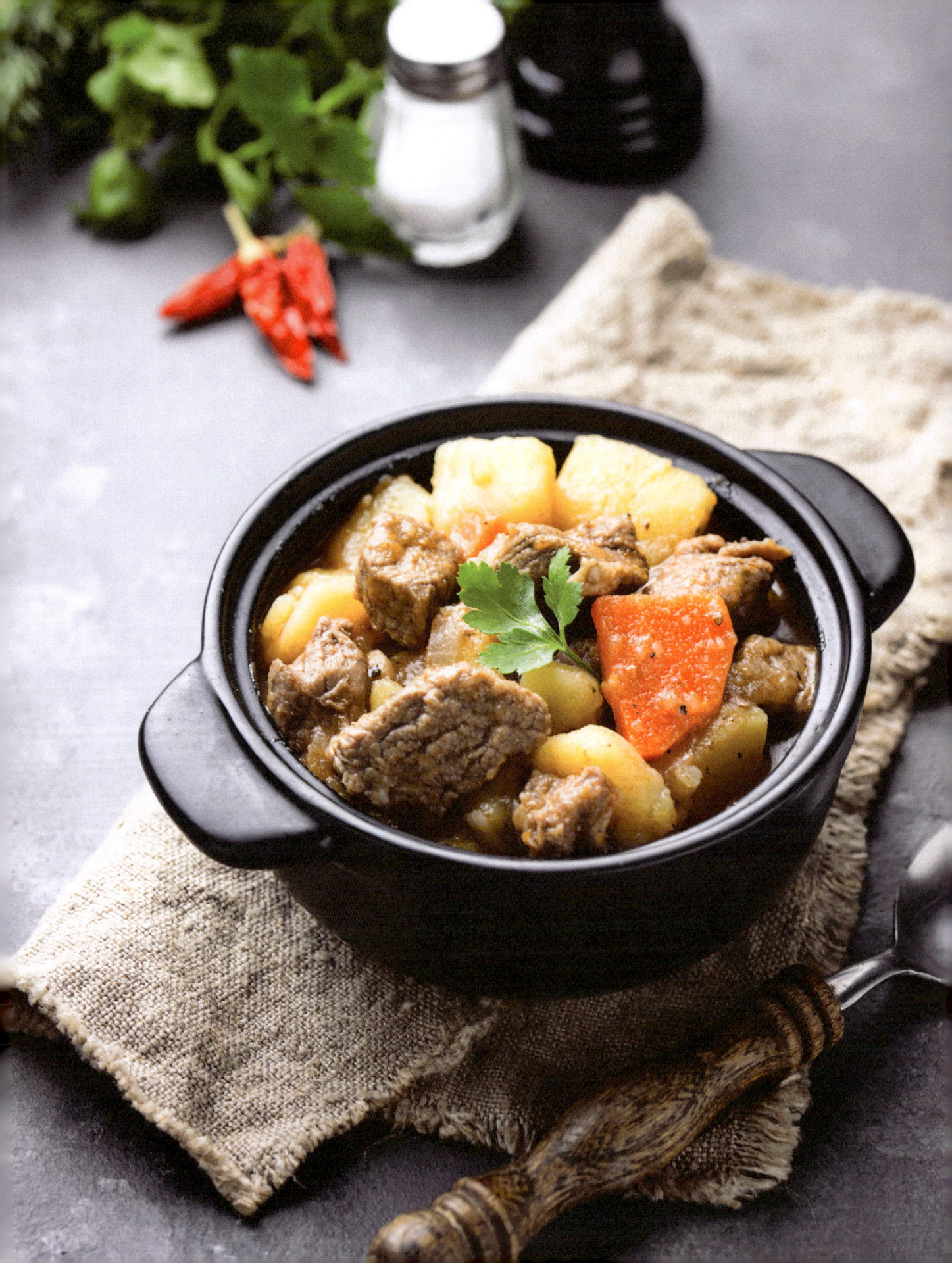

QUICK BEEF STEW   Serves 4

INGREDIENTS:

1 onion, sliced

3 cups beef mince or stew meat

3 garlic cloves, minced

2 cups beef stock

2 tbsp rice flour

1 stick celery, diced

2 tbsp Worcestershire sauce

3 large potatoes, diced

5 carrots, diced

1 1/2 cups tomato passata

2 tbsp coconut oil

Pepper (to taste)

Salt (to taste)

METHOD:

- Salt and pepper the beef. Heat a soup pot with the coconut oil and add the beef. Cook until the outside is lightly browned and then add the onion, celery and garlic.

- Cook until fragrant before pouring in the stock and adding in the potatoes, carrots, passata, Worcestershire sauce and some salt and pepper.

- Stir well and bring to the boil. Next, place the lid on top, reduce the heat to a simmer and then gently cook for around 40 minutes. Stir occasionally.

- Meanwhile, mix the rice flour with a few tbsp of cold water and then add into the pot halfway through cooking.

- Once cooked serve immediately.

OVEN CHEESE & TOMATO CHICKEN — Serves 2

INGREDIENTS:

4 chicken breasts
1 tbsp olive oil
3/4 cup soft goat's cheese
3 large tomatoes, sliced
3 cups mixed salad
1 garlic clove, minced
3 tbsp balsamic vinegar
Pepper (to taste)
Salt (to taste)

METHOD:

- Salt the chicken. Preheat the oven to 180°C. Make a slit in each chicken breast ensuring not to cut all the way through. Mix the goats cheese with the garlic and some black pepper and then spoon into the slits of each chicken breast.

- Place the chicken in an ovenproof dish and then cover each slit with 2 or 3 slices of tomato. Drizzle with the olive oil and then place in the oven for about 30 minutes until the chicken is cooked through.

- Plate the salad, and when the chicken is ready serve alongside it. Drizzle both with the balsamic vinegar (to taste).

- Drizzle over extra olive oil if desired too.

"Food is your body's fuel. Without fuel, your body wants to shut down."

—KEN HILL

SALMON & VEGGIE ROAST — Serves 2-4

INGREDIENTS:

- 4 salmon fillets
- 4 beetroots, peeled, cubed
- 16 cherry tomatoes
- 4 garlic cloves
- 2 cups small potatoes, halved
- 2 lemons, quartered
- 2 red onions, quartered
- 1 brocoli head, trimmed, chopped
- 2 tbsp coconut oil
- Pepper (to taste)
- Salt (to taste)

METHOD:

- Preheat the oven to 200°C.

- Place the potatoes, beetroot and garlic on an oven tray with 1 tbsp coconut oil and some salt and pepper. Cook in the oven for around 25 minutes until turning golden.

- When ready, add the onion, tomatoes, lemon and broccoli to the tray with the remaining coconut oil and some more salt and pepper. Mix around and then nestle the salmon fillets amongst the vegetables.

- Return to the oven for around another 15 minutes until the salmon is done. Serve hot.

OVEN TROUT Serves 2

INGREDIENTS:

4 trout fillets
8 parsley sprigs
2 lemons, sliced
4 cups potatoes, quartered
4 cups spinach

2 tbsp butter
2 tbsp coconut oil
Pepper (to taste)
Salt (to taste)

METHOD:

- Preheat the oven to 180°C. Cut four sheets of baking paper that are bigger than the trout fillets. Rub each fillet with the oil, season with salt and pepper and then lay each fillet skin side down on a sheet of baking paper. Lay lemon slices and parsley sprigs on each fillet. Fold over the baking paper to form small parcels. Place on an oven tray and cook for 10-15 minutes until the trout is done.

- Meanwhile, place the potatoes in a pot of salted water and bring to the boil. Continue to cook for another 15 minutes until softened. On the final minute of cooking add the spinach to the water to wilt it. Drain, and then mash the potatoes together with the spinach. Add in the butter and some more salt and pepper if necessary.

- Plate the mash alongside the trout and serve immediately.

STEAK & SWEET POTATO FRIES — Serves 2

INGREDIENTS:

2 7oz beef steaks
2 tsp rice flour
2 large sweet potatoes
1/2 tsp paprika
1/2 tsp garlic powder

3 tbsp coconut oil
Pepper (to taste)
Salt (to taste)

METHOD:

- Salt and pepper the steaks. Preheat the oven to 200°C.

- Slice the sweet potato into uniformed long batons. In a bowl, mix 2 tbsp coconut oil with the garlic, paprika, rice flour and some salt and pepper.

- Place the fries on a lined oven tray and mix with the coconut oil mixture. Once well combined, place the tray in the oven and cook the fries for about 25 minutes until they are crispy. Mix the fries around halfway through cooking.

- Meanwhile, heat a frying pan with 1 tbsp coconut oil and then add the steaks to the pan. I recommend cooking the steaks to rare which takes about 2 minutes each side. However, you may need to cook them longer for thicker cuts.

- Once done, remove the steaks from the pan and leave to rest for a few minutes. Plate up the steaks alongside the fries and eat hot.

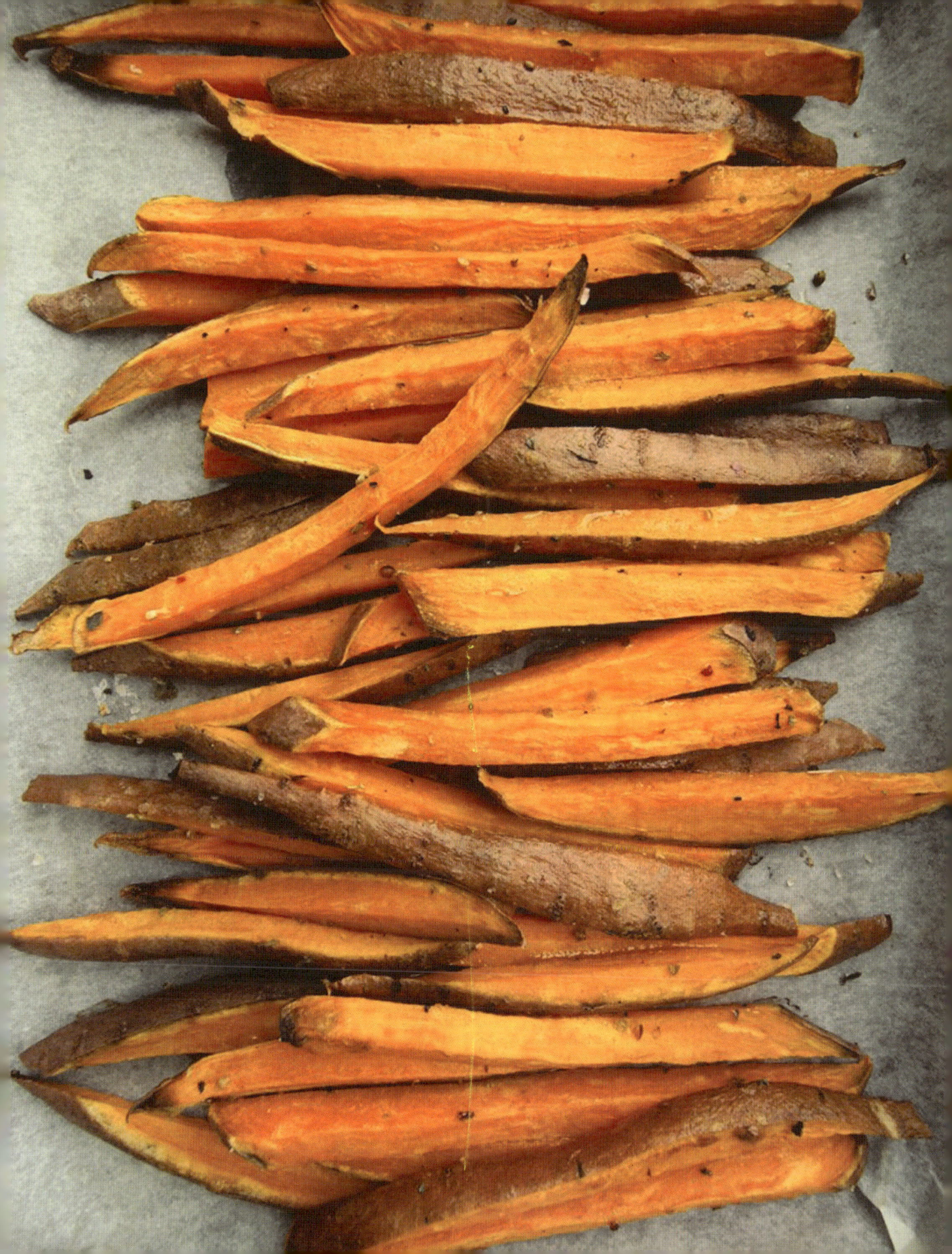

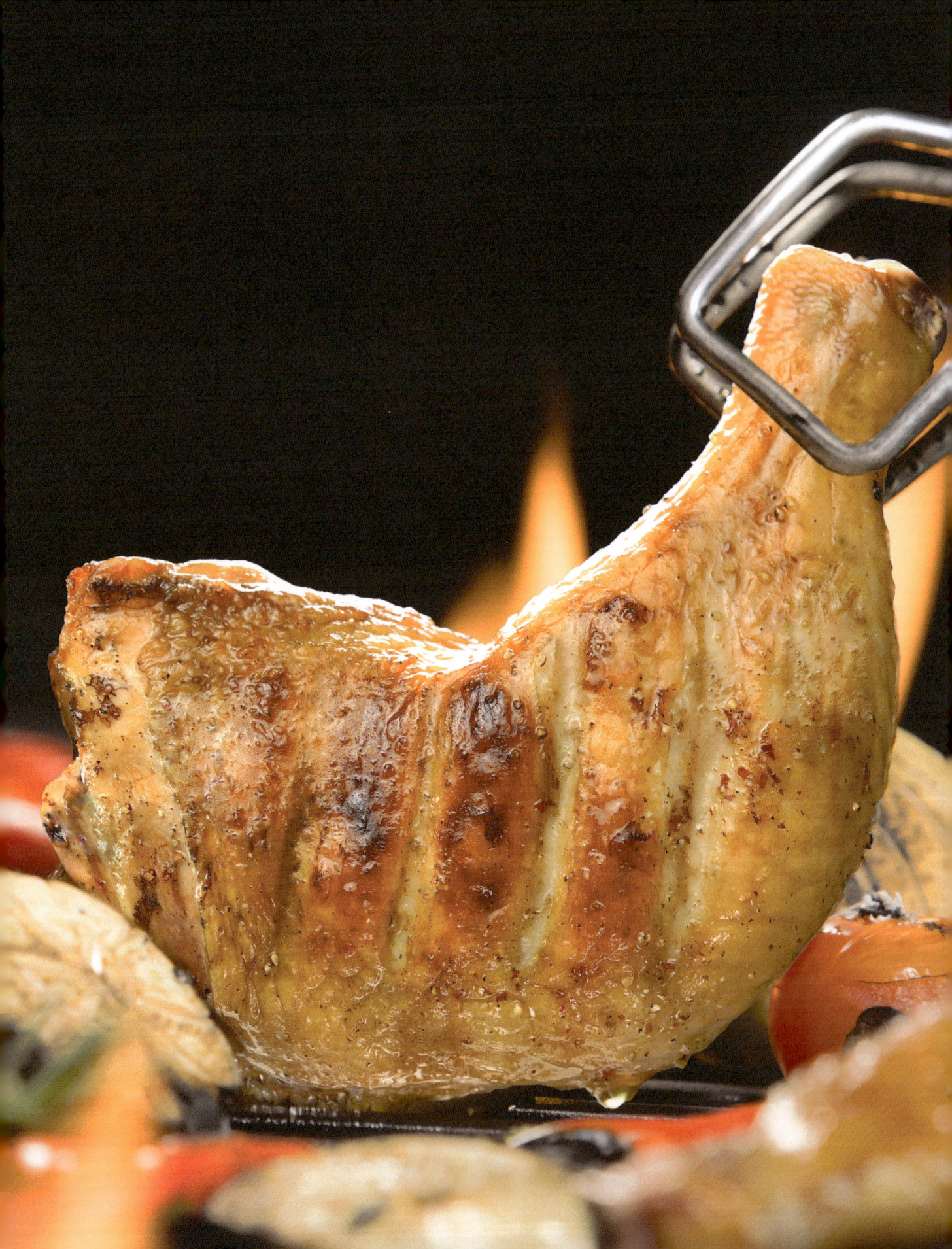

ONEPOT CREAMY CHICKEN DISH   Serves 4

INGREDIENTS:

- 6 chicken thighs
- 3 tbsp coconut oil
- 4 shallots, sliced
- 1 garlic, minced
- 2 cups carrots, diced
- 2 tbsp rice flour
- 1 tbsp Dijon mustard
- 2 cups chicken stock
- 1/2 lemon, juiced
- 1 broccoli head, trimmed, chopped
- 2 cups green beans, trimmed
- 1/2 cup double cream
- 1 tbsp honey
- 1 tbsp parsley, chopped
- 2 cups potatoes, diced
- Pepper (to taste)
- Salt (to taste)

METHOD:

- Salt the chicken. Heat a soup pot with the coconut oil and fry the chicken thighs for about 5 minutes on each side. Set aside and then add in the shallots, garlic, carrots and potatoes. Sprinkle with salt and pepper and then fry for about 5 minutes before adding in the flour, mustard and honey for a further minute.

- Next, pour in the stock and add the chicken back in to the pan. Bring it all to the boil then reduce to a simmer and cover for 15 minutes. Once the time is up, add in the green beans for a further 10 minutes before stirring in the lemon juice, cream and parsley. Turn off the heat and serve hot.

> "You could probably get through life without knowing how to roast a chicken, but the question is, would you want to?"
>
> – NIGELLA LAWSON

EASY LAMB GOULASH Serves 2-4

INGREDIENTS:

4 lamb chops, cut into chunks
3 cups potatoes, diced
2 tsp paprika
1/2 cup yoghurt
1 cup mushrooms, sliced
1 1/2 cups lamb stock

1 tbsp parsley, chopped
1 cup tomato passata
3 tbsp coconut oil
Pepper (to taste)
Salt (to taste)

METHOD:

- Salt and pepper the lamb. Heat a soup pot with coconut oil and then fry the lamb chops in batches for a few minutes until they have browned. Set aside.

- Next, cook the mushrooms in the same pot for a few minutes before adding in the paprika, potatoes, passata and some salt and pepper. Then, pour in enough stock to cover the potatoes. Bring it all to the boil and then reduce to a simmer. Cover with a lid and allow to cook for about 15 minutes until the potatoes have cooked through. Finally, add the lamb to the pan for a further 10 minutes and continue to simmer.

- To serve, plate the goulash and top with the yoghurt and parsley.

NUTRITOUS HEART & RICE STEW

Serves 2

INGREDIENTS:

- 1/2 beef heart, trimmed of excess fat, cubed
- 1 1/2 cups beef stock
- 1/2 tsp paprika
- 1 tsp rice flour
- 1 onion, diced
- 1/2 cup white rice
- 1/2 tsp garlic powder
- 2 tbsp parsley, chopped
- 2 tbsp coconut oil
- Pepper (to taste)
- Salt (to taste)

METHOD:

- Salt and pepper the heart. Heat a soup pot with the coconut oil and then add the heart.
- Fry until browned before adding in the onion. Cook for another few minutes and then add in the stock, paprika, garlic and some more salt and pepper.
- Mix the rice flour with 1 tbsp water and then add into the pot. Bring the stock to the boil and then reduce to a simmer. Cover and allow to gently cook for 60 minutes.
- Once the time is up, pour in the rice and continue to simmer until the rice has fully softened.
- Serve up hot and garnish with the parsley.

TUSCAN SHRIMP & NOODLES — Serves 4

INGREDIENTS:

- 2 cups shrimp, peeled
- 1/4 cup basil, torn
- 1/4 cup Parmesan, grated
- 1 onion, diced
- 1/2 cup double cream
- 2 tbsp coconut oil
- 1 lemon, quartered
- 2 cups rice stick noodles
- 1 1/2 cups cherry tomatoes, halved
- 3 cups spinach
- 3 garlic cloves, minced
- 3 tbsp butter
- Pepper (to taste)
- Salt (to taste)

METHOD:

- Heat a large frying pan with the coconut oil. Add in the garlic and fry for about 1 minute. Next, add in the shrimp and some salt.

- Cook the shrimp until they are pink and just cooked through, around 3 minutes. Set aside.

- Then, add in the butter and onion. Cook for a few minutes until the onion begins to soften and then add in the cherry tomatoes. Add more salt and some pepper. Continue to cook for a further few minutes until the tomatoes begin to soften and then tip in the spinach.

- Once the spinach has wilted, add in the parmesan, cream and basil. Cook for about 5 minutes until the sauce begins to reduce. Finally, stir the shrimp back into the sauce and cook until heated through.

- Meanwhile, bring a pot of water to the boil and add the rice noodles to the water with some salt. Cook for about 3-5 minutes until just soft to bite.

- Drain and serve onto plates, spooning the tuscan shrimp dish on top. Serve with the lemon wedges.

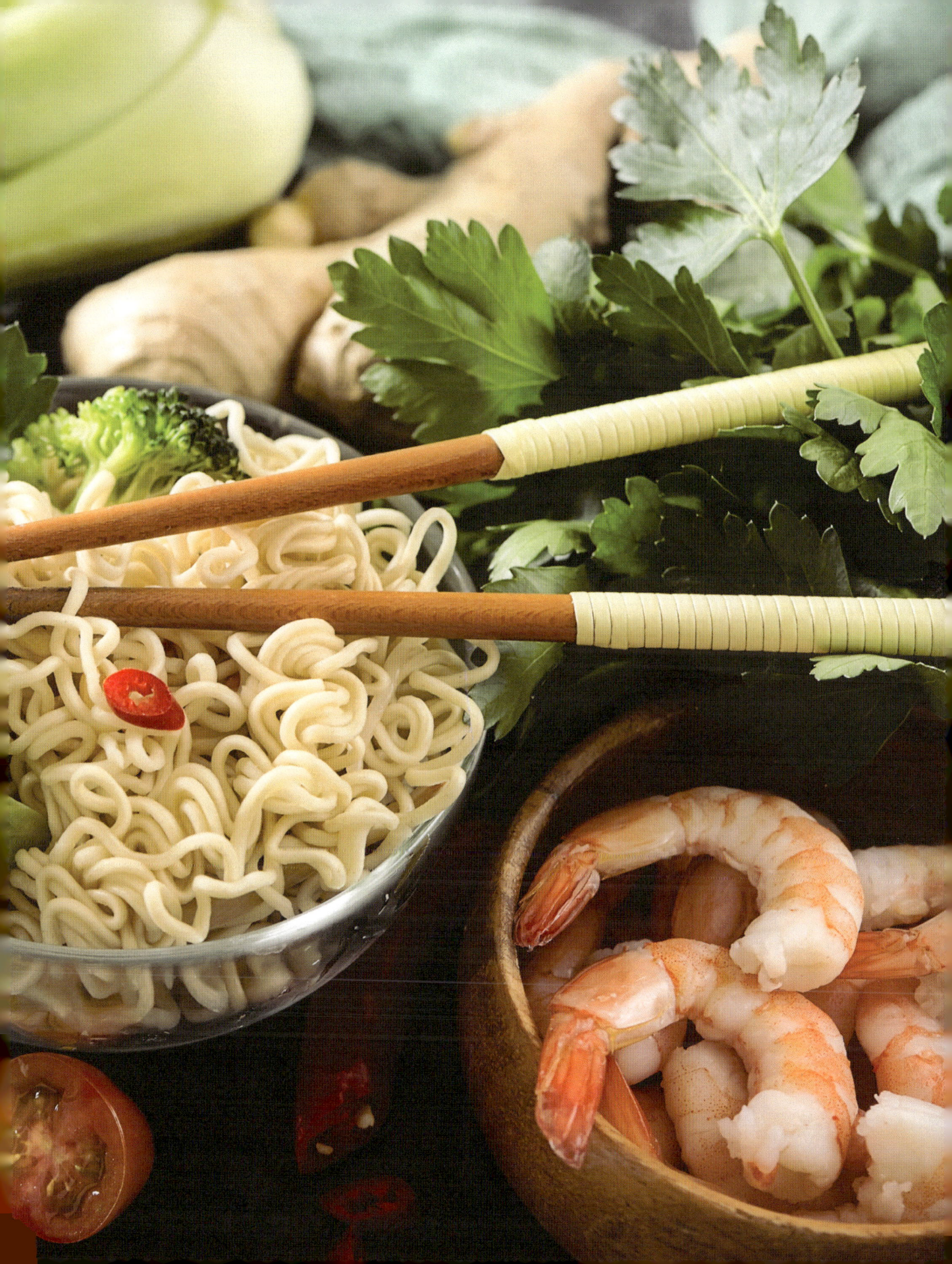

"I know that once people get connected to <u>real</u> food, they never change back."

—ALICE WATERS

FAST CHEESY MINCE & TATTIES   Serves 2-4

INGREDIENTS:

2 1/2 cups beef mince
1 1/2 cups cheese, grated
3 cups potatoes, peeled
2 tbsp milk
1 tbsp coconut oil

Pepper (to taste)
Salt (to taste)

METHOD:

- Salt the mince. Place the potatoes in a pot and fill with water. Add a generous helping of salt to the water and then put the pot on a medium heat. Bring to the boil and cook for a further 10-15 minutes until the potatoes are soft all the way through. To check this, poke the largest one with a fork-it should slide into the potato with little resistance. When done, drain and set aside.

- Meanwhile, heat a frying pan with the coconut oil and then add the mince with some salt and pepper. Cook until browned and fully cooked. Turn off the heat and then add in the grated cheese.

- Next, mash up the potatoes with the milk until a thick, silky mash forms. Add more salt and pepper if desired. Serve hot with the mince.

ROASTED CHICKEN RATATOUILLE

Serves 2-4

INGREDIENTS:

2 red onions, cut into wedges
3 garlic cloves, minced
2 red peppers, seeded, cubed
1 aubergine, cubed
1 courgette, cut into half moons
1 tbsp balsamic vinegar
4 large tomatoes, quartered
4 chicken thighs, skin on

3 tbsp olive oil
1/2 lemon, zested
2 cups tomato passata
1 tbsp honey
1 tbsp basil leaves, torn
Pepper (to taste)
Salt (to taste)

METHOD:

- Salt and pepper the chicken. Preheat the oven to 180°C. Lay the tomatoes, courgette, aubergine and onion on an oven tray. Sprinkle with salt and pepper. Top with the chicken thighs and drizzle the whole tray with the olive oil. Cook in the oven for 15-20 minutes.

- Meanwhile, mix the passata with the garlic, honey, balsamic vinegar and some salt and pepper. Once the time is up, pour the passata mix into the tray and coat the vegetables and chicken with it. Place the tray back in the oven for another 15 minutes until the vegetables and chicken are cooked. If the passata gets too thick, you can loosen it with some added water.

- Once done, add in the zest to taste and the basil leaves. Mix well and serve hot.

PIQUANT COD & YAMS   Serves 2-4

INGREDIENTS:

4 cod fillets
6 tbsp chives, chopped
2 tbsp coconut oil
3 tbsp olive oil
1 lemon, zested, juiced
4 yams, peeled, cubed

1 cup frozen peas
2 tbsp capers, chopped
3 cups rocket
Pepper (to taste)
Salt (to taste)

METHOD:

- Salt the cod. Place the yams in a pot of salted water, bring to the boil and continue to cook for 15 minutes until softened. In the final 2 minutes of cooking, add the peas. Roughly crush together into a chunky mash. Stir in 1 tbsp olive oil, some pepper and more salt, if desired.

- Meanwhile, mix the remaining olive oil, capers, chives, lemon juice and zest and some salt and pepper in a bowl.

- Next, heat a frying pan with the coconut oil and fry the cod fillets for a few minutes on each side until cooked. Serve alongside the chunky mash and rocket. Top the fish with the dressing.

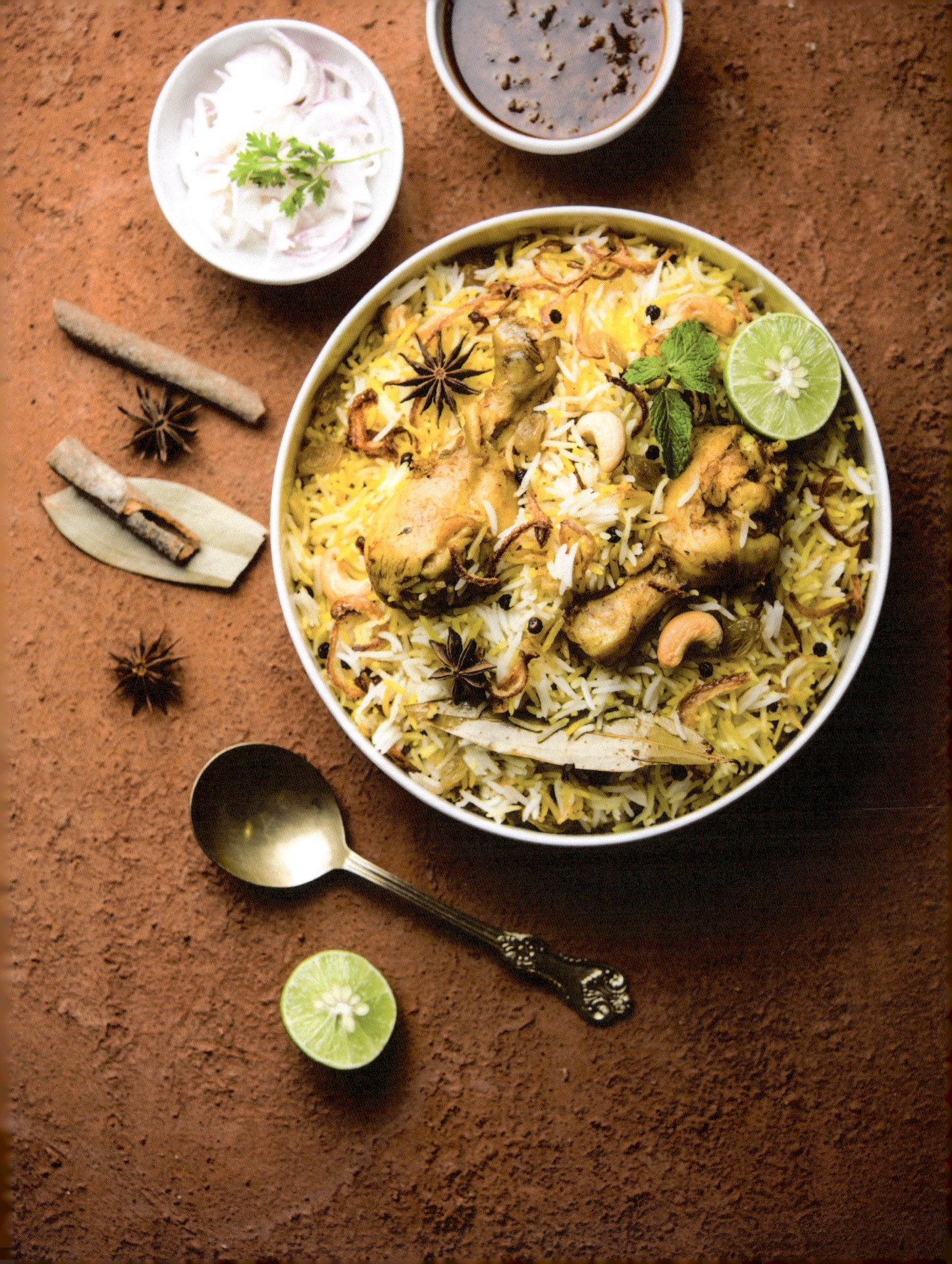

BASIC CHICKEN BIRYANI   Serves 4

INGREDIENTS:

5 chicken thighs, quartered
1 1/2 cups rice
1 red onion, sliced
2 cups peas
2 tbsp curry powder
1 bay leaf

2 tbsp butter
3 cups chicken stock
2 tbsp coriander, chopped
Cashew nuts (to decorate)
2 lime wedges, halved
Salt (to taste)

METHOD:

- Salt the chicken. Heat the butter in a soup pot and then fry the onion and bay leaf for around 5 minutes.

- Next, add the chicken thigh chunks, and the curry powder. Cook for 2 minutes before adding in the stock and rice. Bring it all to the boil and simmer for 6 minutes.

- Pour in the peas for the final 30 seconds and then turn off the heat. Place the lid on the pan and let it sit for at least 10 minutes until all the stock has been absorbed and the rice and chicken are cooked.

- When done, stir in the coriander and add more salt if desired.

- Serve hot with cashew nuts sprinkled on top and the lime halves.

"The main facts in human life are five: birth, food, sleep, love and death."

– E.M. FORSTER

PORK & APPLE RICE BOWL   Serves 2

INGREDIENTS:

3 cups pork mince

1 tbsp honey

1 large apple, cored, diced

1 onion, diced

1 tbsp parsley, chopped

2 tbsp coconut oil

1 tbsp wholegrain mustard

1 cup rice

Pepper (to taste)

Salt (to taste)

METHOD:

- Salt the mince. Boil a pot of salted water. Rinse the rice under cold water to remove any excess starch and then place in the boiling water. Cook for about 15 minutes until it is soft.

- Meanwhile, heat a frying pan with the coconut oil. Tip in the mince and fry for 5 minutes until slightly browned. Then add the onion and cook for a further 5 minutes until it has softened.

- Next, add the mustard, cook for a few minutes and then add in the honey and apple to the pan. Continue to cook until the mince is cooked through and the apple is beginning to caramelise.

- Once done, stir the parsley through the mince. Spoon the rice into bowls and top with the mince.

SMOKY BBQ MEATBALLS WITH RICE & PAK CHOI   Serves 2

INGREDIENTS:

- 2 pak choi
- 1 1/4 cups beef mince
- 1 egg
- 1/3 cup rice flour
- 1/2 red onion, finely chopped
- 2 tbsp Worcestershire sauce
- 2 tbsp balsamic vinegar
- 2 tbsp honey
- 1/2 tsp paprika
- 4 tbsp tomato puree
- 1/2 cup white rice
- 2 spring onions, sliced
- Pepper (to taste)
- Salt (to taste)

METHOD:

- Preheat the oven to 180°C. Mix together the beef, egg, flour and red onion with some salt and pepper. Shape into meatballs and cook on an oven tray rack for 40 minutes.

- Meanwhile, boil a pot of salted water and blanch the pak choi for 45 seconds. Once done, set aside. Now, add the rice to the boiling water and cook until soft (about 10-15 minutes). Once done, drain and set aside.

- To make the sauce, combine the tomato puree, paprika, honey, vinegar, Worcestershire sauce, and some pepper and salt. Heat up in a pan for about 3 minutes.

- To serve up, spoon the rice onto the plate and arrange the meatballs and pak choi on top. Then pour over the sauce and enjoy!

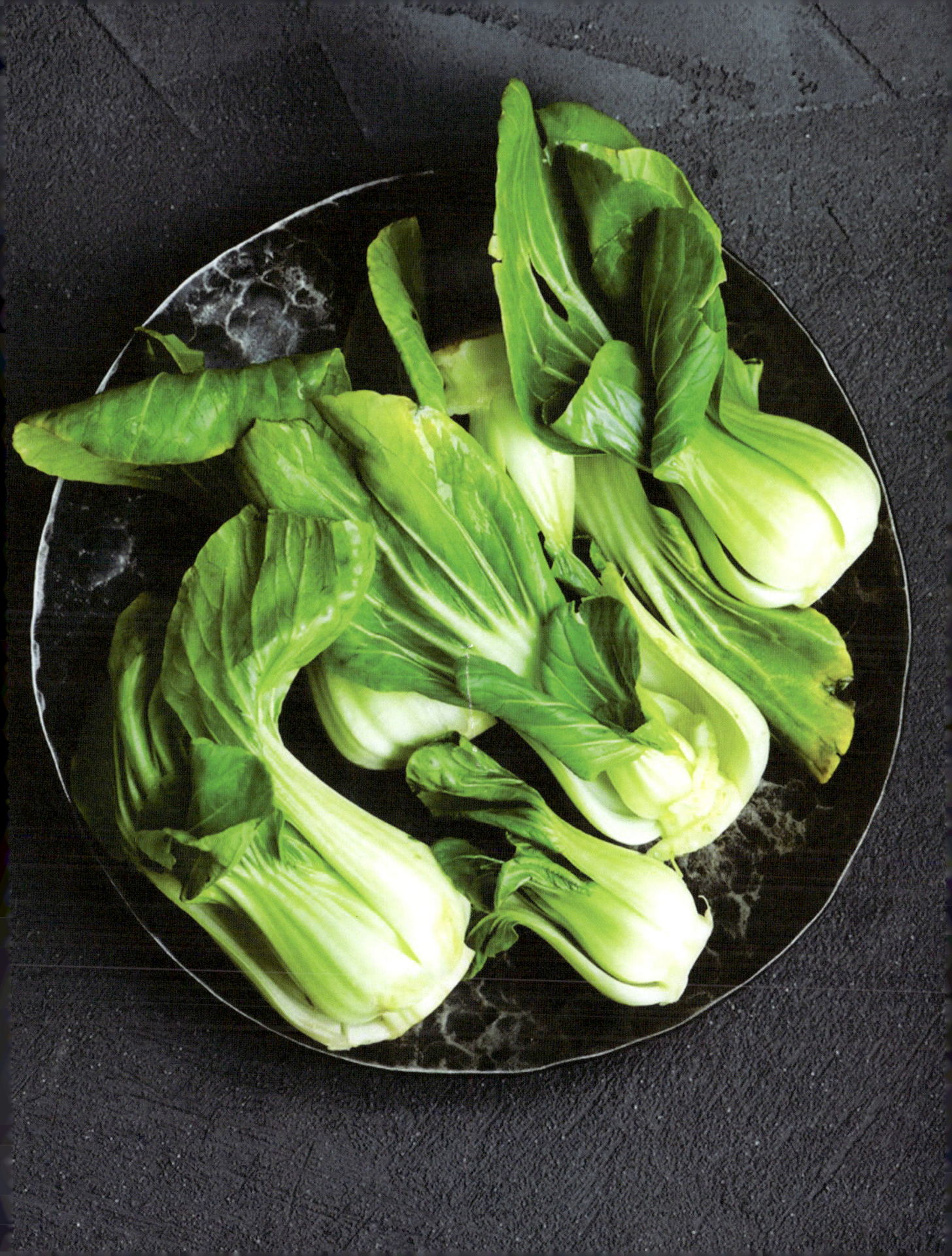

CHICKEN CURRY WITH POTATO & SQUASH   Serves 2-4

INGREDIENTS:

2 cups baby potatoes
1 cup chicken stock
1 bell pepper, seeded, diced
2 tbsp coconut oil
1 can of thick coconut milk
1 onion, sliced
1 cup tomatoes, chopped
3 chicken breasts, cubed
2 tbsp curry powder
2 garlic cloves, minced
4 tbsp fresh ginger, minced
2 tbsp tomato puree
3 cups butternut squash, peeled, seeded, cubed
8 sprigs of fresh coriander, chopped
Salt (to taste)

METHOD

- Preheat the oven to 200°C. Salt the diced chicken breasts. Add the potatoes to an oven tray with 1 tbsp coconut oil and some salt. Cook for about 30 minutes until the potatoes are soft and golden. Meanwhile, heat up a large frying pan with the remaining coconut oil and then add in the chicken.

- Once the outside of the chicken is no longer pink, add the squash to the pan. After 5 minutes add in the onion, garlic, ginger, pepper and curry powder. Once the onions start to soften and the spices and other aromatics have started to give off a nice smell, pour in the stock, coconut milk, tomatoes and tomato puree. Sprinkle in more salt.

- Simmer the curry for around 15 minutes. If the sauce thickens too much then loosen with water. Add in the potatoes and coriander once the curry is ready and the chicken has been fully cooked.

SEARED STEAK WITH 'MUSTARDY' MASH

Serves 2

INGREDIENTS:

- 2 large potatoes, diced
- 2 7oz beef steaks
- 2 carrots, diagonally sliced
- 2 parsnips, diagonally sliced
- 2 tsp mustard
- 2 tbsp balsamic vinegar
- 1 tbsp honey
- 1 tbsp fresh chives, chopped
- 1 1/4 cups beef stock
- 1 1/2 cups kale, torn
- 1 tsp gelatin powder
- 3 tbsp cranberry sauce
- 2 tbsp coconut oil
- 1 tbsp butter
- 1 1/3 cups beetroot, peeled, cut into wedges
- Pepper (to taste)
- Salt (to taste)

METHOD:

- Preheat the oven to 200°C. Season the steaks with salt and pepper. Bring a pot of water to the boil. Add in the potatoes and some salt. Cook for 15 minutes until soft, then drain and mash.

- Add the carrots, beetroot and parsnips to an oven tray and toss with 1 tbsp of coconut oil, salt and pepper. Toast for around 25 minutes until cooked.

- Meanwhile, heat a frying pan with the remaining coconut oil. Sear the steaks and cook to your desired level (2 minutes each side for rare, 5 minutes each side for well done). Once done, remove from the pan, and cook the kale in the steak fat and juices until wilted. Set aside when done.

- Finally, mix the stock, cranberry sauce, gelatin, honey and cranberry sauce mix. Heat up in the frying pan for 5 minutes. Add more water if needed. To finish the potatoes, add in the butter, chives, vinegar, kale and some salt. Slice the steak and serve up!

TANGY TURKEY & STUFFED PEPPERS

Inspired by **EndoBoss® Alumni** - Rachel Sledge from USA

Serves 2

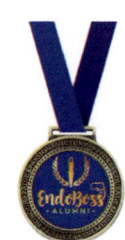

INGREDIENTS:

4 bell peppers
1 cup courgette, diced
1 cup onion, diced
2 cups turkey mince
1 cup brown rice
1 tsp chilli powder
2 tbsp cider vinegar
2 tbsp brown mustard

1 garlic clove, minced
2 tbsp Worcestershire sauce
2 tbsp honey
2/3 cup tomato passata
1/3 cup molasses
2 cups vegetable stock
Pepper (to taste)
Salt (to taste)

METHOD:

- To make the BBQ sauce, combine the chilli powder, vinegar, mustard, tomato paste, honey and molasses with some salt and pepper in a pan. Bring to the boil and simmer for 2 minutes. Set aside when done.

- Preheat the oven to 180°C. Cut off the tops off the peppers, clean out the seeds and set them aside. Combine the onion, garlic, courgette and turkey mince in a pot and gently fry with 1 tbsp of olive oil and some salt until partly cooked. Next, add in the vegetable stock, rice and BBQ sauce (to taste). Cook on a medium heat for around 30 minutes.

- Once the mixture is cooked pour the mixture into the peppers and bake for 20-30 minutes.

SAVOURY MINCE & CAULIFLOWER RICE   Serves 2

INGREDIENTS:

- 1 medium cauliflower, cut into small florets
- 2 cups beef mince
- 2 tsp oregano
- 2 cups of beef stock
- 2 garlic cloves
- 1 tsp Worcestershire sauce
- 1 cup frozen mixed veg
- 3 tbsp tomato puree
- 1 tbsp coconut oil
- 1 large red onion, diced
- Salt (to taste)

METHOD:

- Salt the mince. Heat a large frying pan with the coconut oil. Add in the onion and garlic and cook for 2 minutes before gradually adding in the mince. Cook until browned.
- Meanwhile, boil a pot of salted water and add in the cauliflower. Cook for about 20 minutes or until softened. Drain and then mash.
- Once the mince is ready, add in the oregano, tomato puree, stock and Worcestershire sauce. Sprinkle in more salt if needed.
- Cook on a very gentle heat for 15 minutes and then add in the frozen veg, cooking for another 5-10 minutes.
- Serve up by plating the cauliflower rice and then topping with the mince.

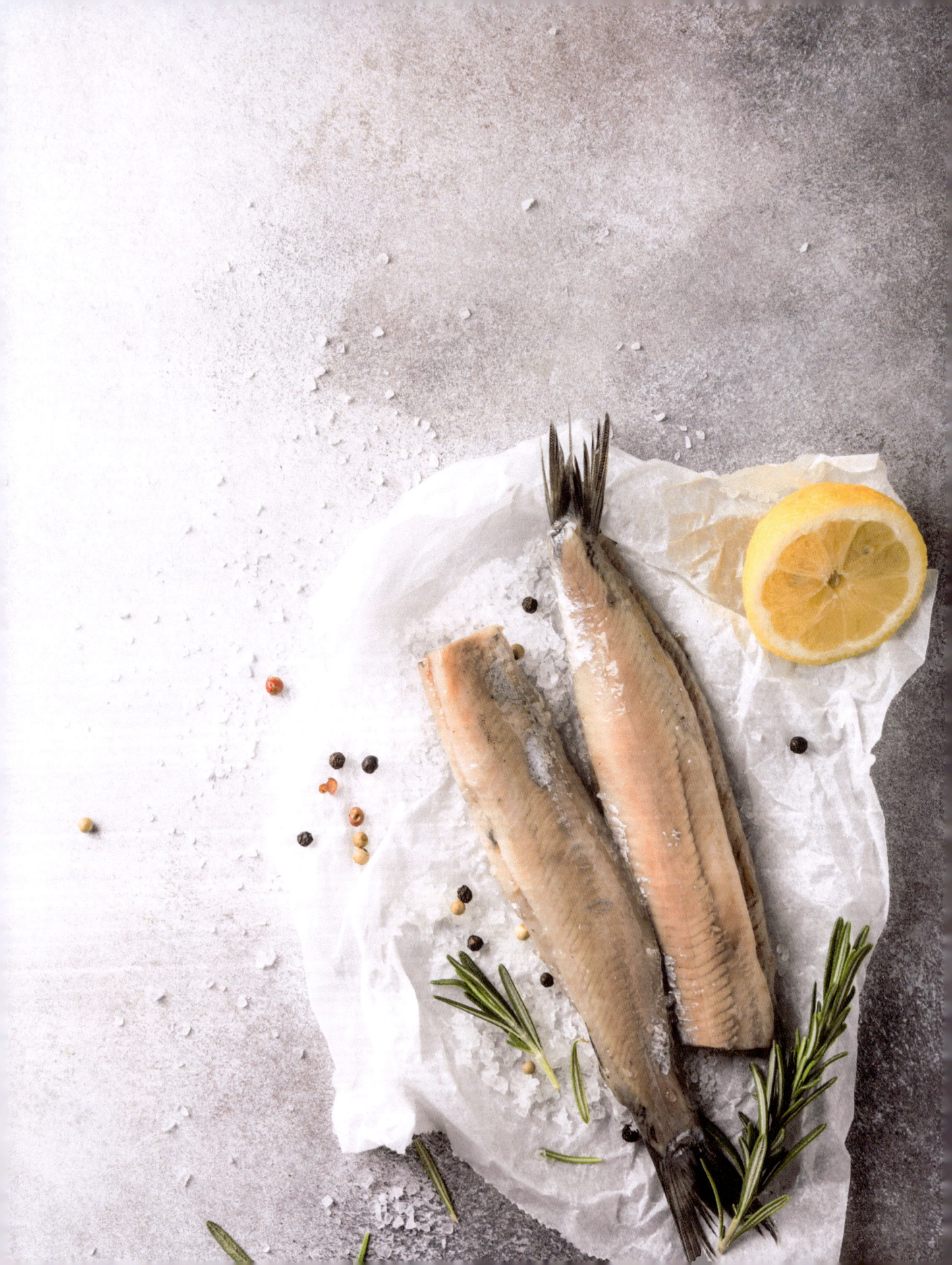

HONEY-MUSTARD HERRING & LEMON RICE   Serves 2

INGREDIENTS:

4 herring fillets
3 tbsp olive oil
1 tbsp wholegrain mustard
3 tbsp basil, torn
1 lemon, zested, juiced
1 tbsp honey

1 1/2 cups Arborio rice
2 eggs
3/4 cup Parmesan, grated
2 tbsp butter
Pepper (to taste)
Salt (to taste)

METHOD:

- Salt the herring fillets. Bring a pot of 7 1/2 cups water to the boil. Heavily salt the water and then pour the rice in. Cook for about 10 minutes until it has softened but still has a bite. Once done, drain the rice, making sure to reserve 1 cup of the water.

- Meanwhile, whisk the eggs and mix in the lemon juice and zest to taste, and some salt and pepper. When the rice has been drained, gradually whisk the egg mixture into the rice water, being careful not to scramble the eggs.

- Gently reheat the pan with the rice and pour in the egg-water mix, parmesan, butter and some more salt and pepper. Cook for a few minutes until very creamy.

- Next, heat a frying pan with 1 tbsp olive and then fry the fillets for 3-4 minutes on each side until they are cooked.

- To make the dressing for the herring, mix together the basil, honey, mustard, remaining olive oil and some salt and pepper. Pour over the fillets before plating alongside the rice. Serve immediately.

SHRIMPS IN TOMATO SAUCE WITH NOODLES Serves 2-4

INGREDIENTS:

3 1/2 cups shrimps,
1/2 cup tomato passata
1 onion, diced
2 tbsp olive oil
1 garlic clove
1/3 cup black olives, pitted, halved

1 tsp fresh parsley
1 large tomato, chopped
2 cups rice stick noodles
Pepper (to taste)
Salt (to taste)

METHOD:

- Heat a frying pan with the olive oil. Add to the pan the shrimp, onion, garlic and some salt and black pepper. Cook for around 5 minutes and then remove the shrimps and set aside.

- Then, add in the passata, tomatoes, parsley, olives and some more salt and pepper. Cook for around 15 minutes and then add in the shrimp for the final minute of cooking.

- Meanwhile, bring a pot of water to the boil and add the rice noodles to the water with some salt. Cook for about 3-5 minutes until just soft to bite. Drain and serve onto plates, spooning the shrimps in tomato sauce on top.

"Salt is born of the purest of parents: the sun and the sea."

— PYTHAGORAS

"One of the very nicest things about life is the way we must regularly stop whatever it is we are doing and devote our attention to eating."

–LUCIANO PAVAROTTI

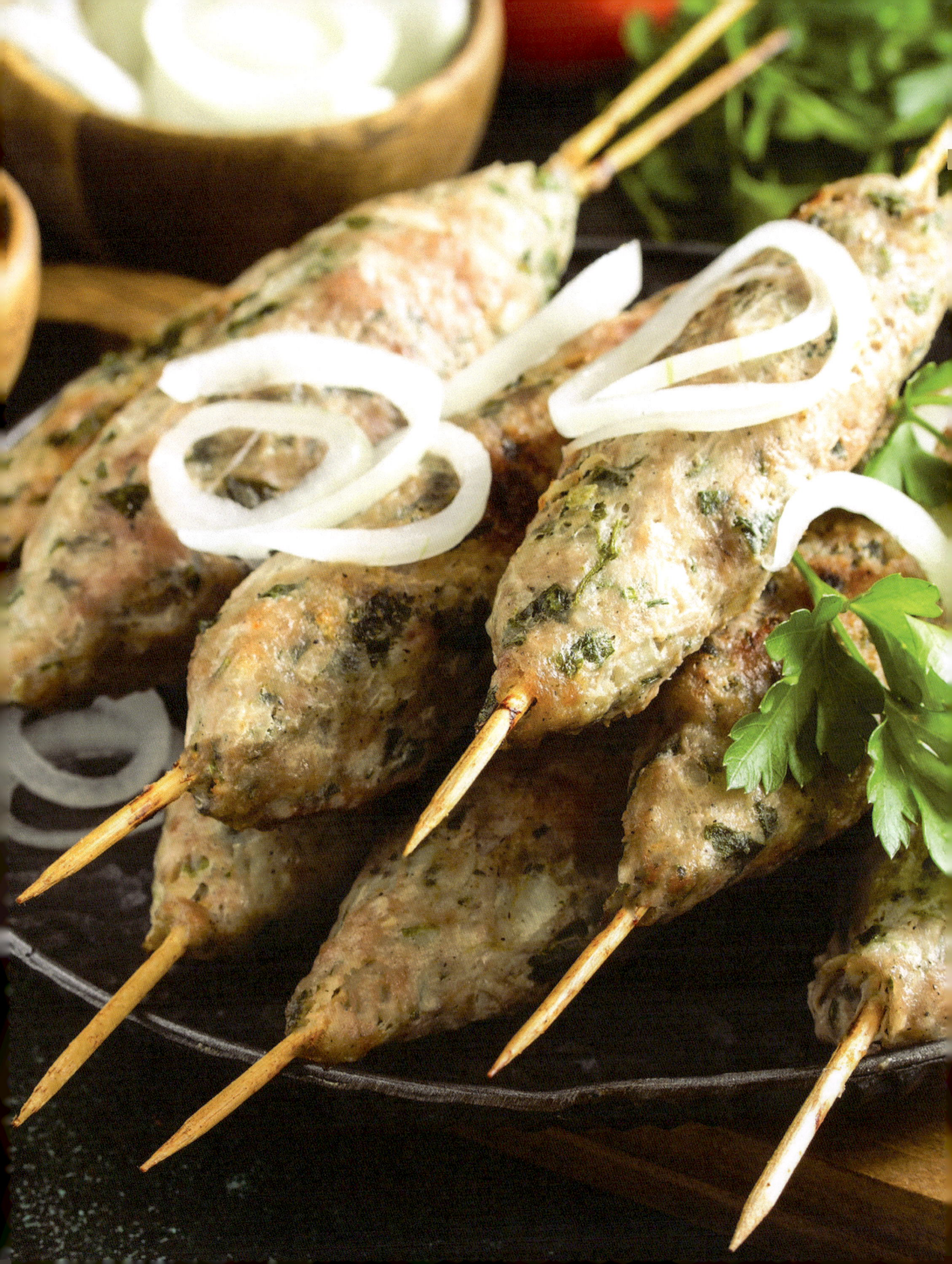

TURKEY KEBABS WITH RED PEPPER GANOUSH   Serves 2

INGREDIENTS:

1 aubergine, halved length ways

1 red bell pepper, halved, seeds and core removed

2 cups turkey mince

1 onion, finely diced

2 tbsp rice flour

1 tsp cumin

6 tbsp olive oil

1 garlic clove, minced

1/2 lemon, juiced

2 tbsp chopped parsley

Pepper (to taste)

Salt (to taste)

METHOD:

- Soak 6 wooden skewers in water. Preheat the oven to 200°C. Place the aubergine halves on an oven tray and brush with 1 tbsp of olive oil. Cook for 10 minutes and then, after brushing that too with oil, add the red pepper to the tray. Cook for around another 15 minutes. You may need to turn the veg as it cooks. Once soft and slightly charred, remove from the oven and set aside.

- Meanwhile, combine the mince with 2 tbsp of olive oil, the flour, garlic, cumin, onion and some salt and pepper. Then form 6 kebabs on the wooden skewers. Place on an oven tray grill and cook for about 25 minutes, or until cooked through and golden on the outside.

- To make the ganoush, remove the skin from both the eggplant and pepper. Squeeze some of the water out of the eggplant. Then, mash both of the veg together with the lemon juice, parsley, 3 tbsp of olive oil and some salt and pepper until fully combined. Serve with the kebabs and enjoy.

HOMEMADE PESTO CHICKEN & HASSELBACK POTATOES   Serves 2

INGREDIENTS:

- 2 cups medium potatoes
- 3 cups fresh basil, torn
- 2 cups asparagus
- 1/3 cup grated parmesan
- 5 tbsp olive oil
- 3 garlic cloves, minced
- 2 chicken breasts
- 1 cup cherry tomatoes
- 1/2 lemon, juiced
- Salt (to taste)

METHOD:

- Preheat the oven to 200°C. Salt the chicken breasts and cut slits in the top of the meat. To make the pesto, crush the basil and garlic into a paste in a pestle and mortar. Add some salt, lemon juice and the parmesan. Next, gradually add in about 2-3 tbsp of olive oil until you have a fluid paste. In an ovenproof dish add the chicken breasts and spoon the pesto on top and into the slits. Roast until cooked through (about 30 minutes).

- Score the potatoes by slicing into them whilst making sure not to cut all the way through. Do this in about 3 mm intervals and travel the width of the potato. Place them in an oven tray, drizzled with 1 tbsp olive oil and sprinkled with salt. Cook until golden and soft.

- Meanwhile, place the tomatoes and asparagus in another tray. Toss with 1 tbsp olive oil and salt. Roast for around 15 minutes until cooked.

- Plate everything together and enjoy!

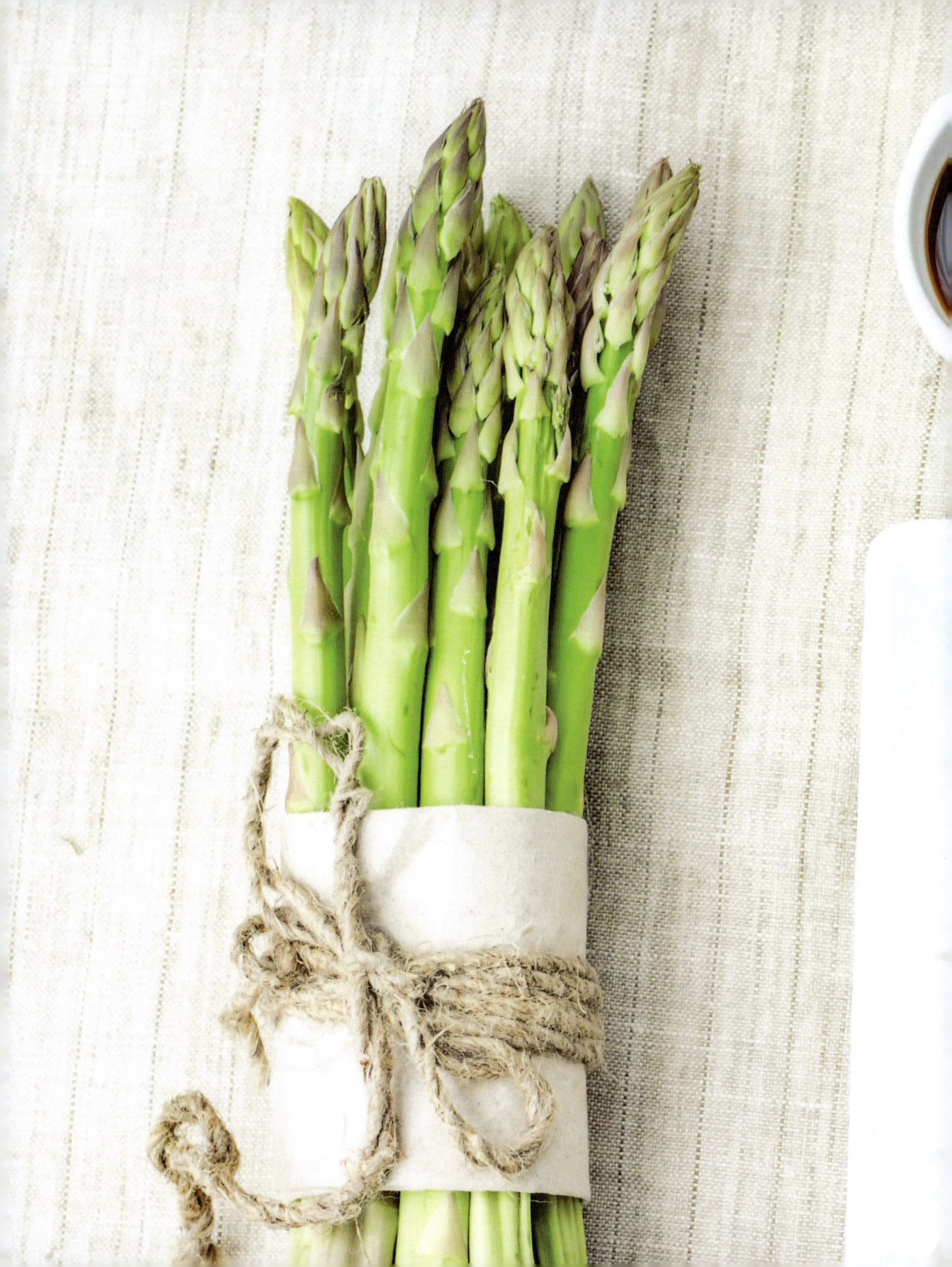

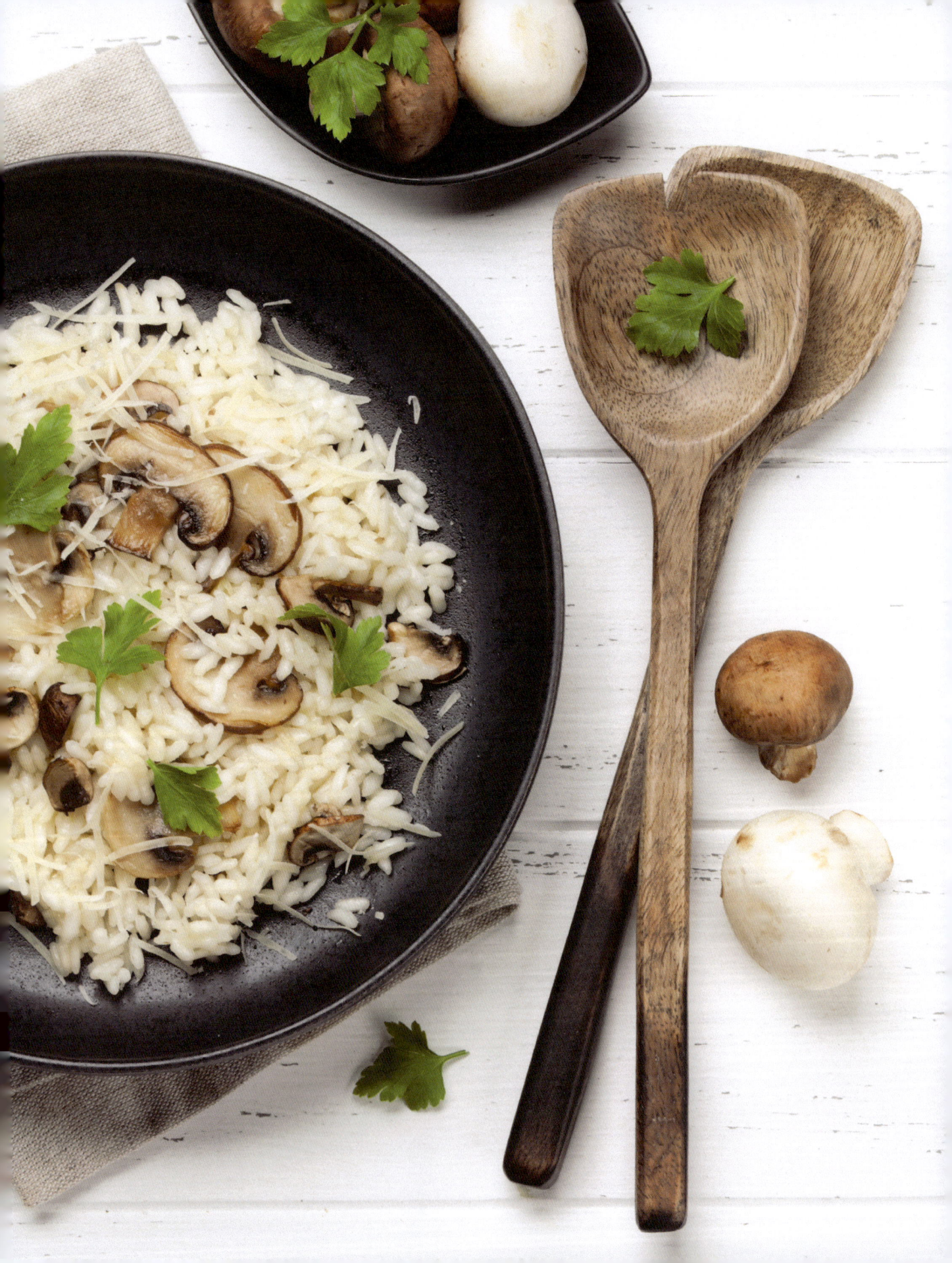

CREAMY MUSHROOM, CHICKEN & BACON RISOTTO

Serves 2

INGREDIENTS:

- 6 rashers of bacon, chopped
- 1 onion, finely chopped
- 2 tbsp parsley, chopped
- 1/2 cup parmesan, grated
- 3/4 cup Arborio rice
- 2 tbsp butter
- 2 cups chestnut mushrooms
- 2 1/2 cups chicken stock
- 1 1/2 cups cooked chicken, torn
- Salt (to taste)

METHOD:

- Fry the bacon and onion in 1 tbsp butter and some salt. Then, when the onion has softened, add the mushrooms and cook until they are soft. Next, pour in the stock with the rice and continue to cook until the rice has softened.

- Finally, add in the chicken and cook for a few minutes before removing the pan from the heat. At this point, add in the parmesan, remaining butter, parsley and some pepper. Mix well and then serve immediately.

"Fish, to taste right, must swim three times – in water, in butter, and in wine."

– POLISH PROVERB

PORK AND APPLE SAUSAGES & CARAMELISED ONIONS WITH PARSNIP & CARROT MASH Serves 2

INGREDIENTS:

6 pork and apple sausages
4 large carrots, sliced
4 large parsnips, sliced
2 tbsp butter
2 red onions, sliced

2 tbsp brown sugar
1 tbsp coconut oil
2 tbsp balsamic vinegar
Pepper (to taste)
Salt (to taste)

METHOD:

- Preheat the oven to 200°C. Boil a pot of water and add to it the carrots, parsnips and some salt. Cook until the veg is tender (about 15 minutes).

- Meanwhile, place the sausages on an oven tray grill and cook for around 25 minutes, until they are cooked through and golden.

- When the parsnips and carrots are cooked, mash them with the butter, and some salt and pepper.

- Finally, in a frying pan, heat up the coconut oil. Then, add the onions with some salt. Cook until very soft, adding some water if the onions start to stick to the pan. Next, add in the balsamic vinegar and the sugar and simmer until a sticky mixture has formed.

- Serve up the sausages with the mash to one side and the onions poured on top.

SHREDDED TOMATO CHICKEN WITH GNOCCHI   Serves 2-4

INGREDIENTS:

1 tsp gelatin powder
4 large potatoes
2 tbsp butter
4 chicken thighs
1 onion, diced
1 tbsp honey
2 tbsp olive oil
1 tbsp coconut oil

4 cups tomatoes, chopped
1 cup tomato paste
2 cloves garlic, minced
2 tbsp basil, chopped
1 cup rice flour
Pepper (to taste)
Salt (to taste)

METHOD:

- Salt the chicken thighs. Preheat the oven to 200°C. Place the potatoes on an oven tray and roast for about 50 minutes or until very tender. Place the chicken thighs in an ovenproof dish with the coconut oil and roast in the oven until cooked through (about 25 minutes).

- Meanwhile, heat the olive oil in a pan and add the onion and garlic for 5 minutes. Then add in the tomato, tomato paste, basil, honey, and some salt and pepper. Stir well and cook until simmering. Turn off the heat and set aside.

- When the potatoes are ready, remove the skin and mash the flesh until very smooth. Combine with the butter and some salt. Cover and chill until no longer warm.

- Whilst the potato is cooling, shred the cooked chicken with two forks. Set aside.

- When no longer warm add in the gelatin and flour to the potato mixture. Begin to knead the mixture together, adding more flour if the dough does not hold together. Be careful not to make it too dry though.

- Next, roll the dough into long cylinders on a lightly floured surface and then leave to sit for 5 minutes. Meanwhile, boil a pot of water and keep simmering. Then, cut the dough into smaller 1 inch-long cylinders. Indent the gnocchi with the back of a fork. Once ready, drop half into the boiling water, cooking for 3 minutes before removing and repeating with the other half.

- Plate the gnocchi before topping with the shredded chicken and pouring over the tomato sauce. Garnish with more basil if desired.

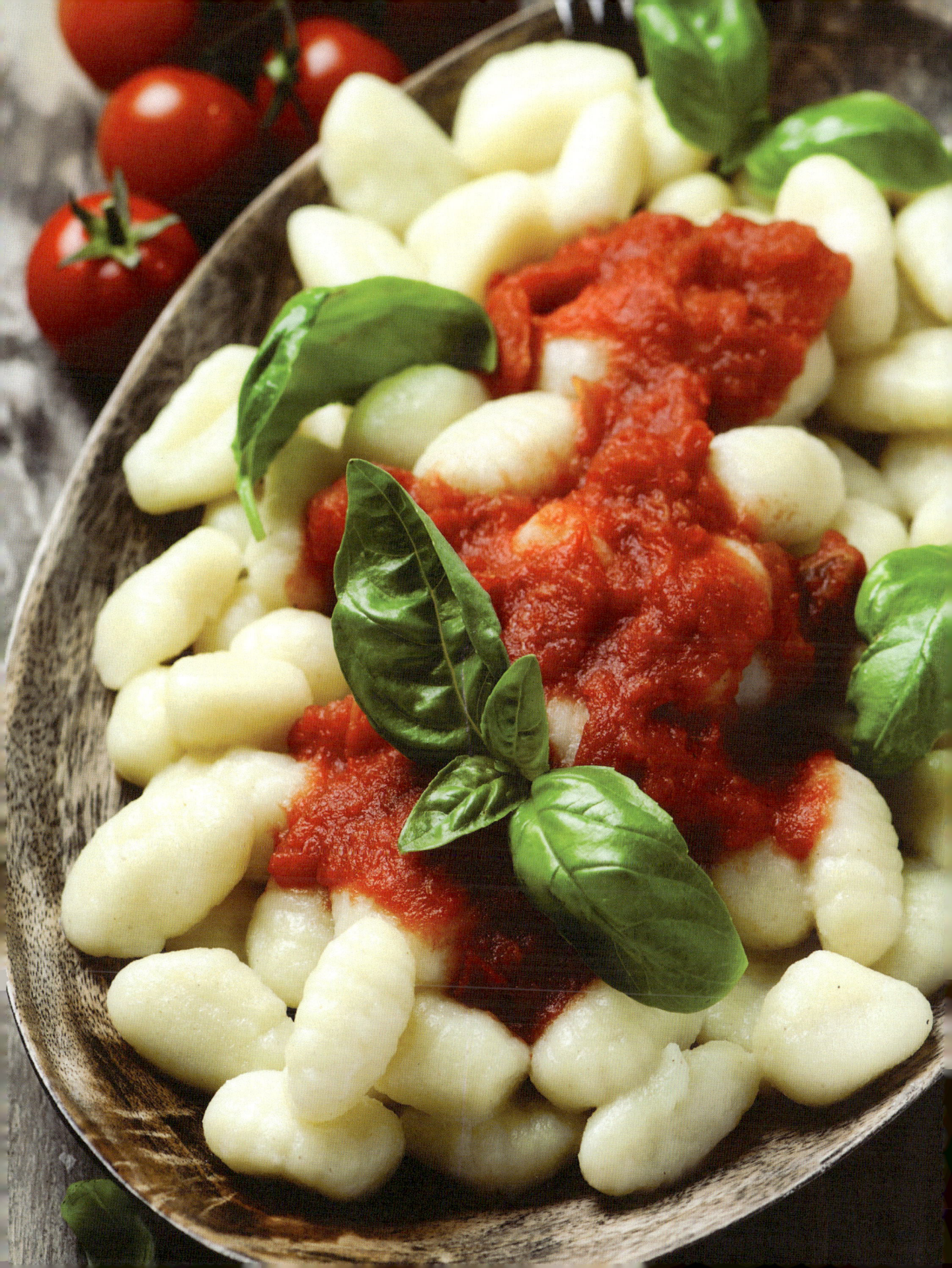

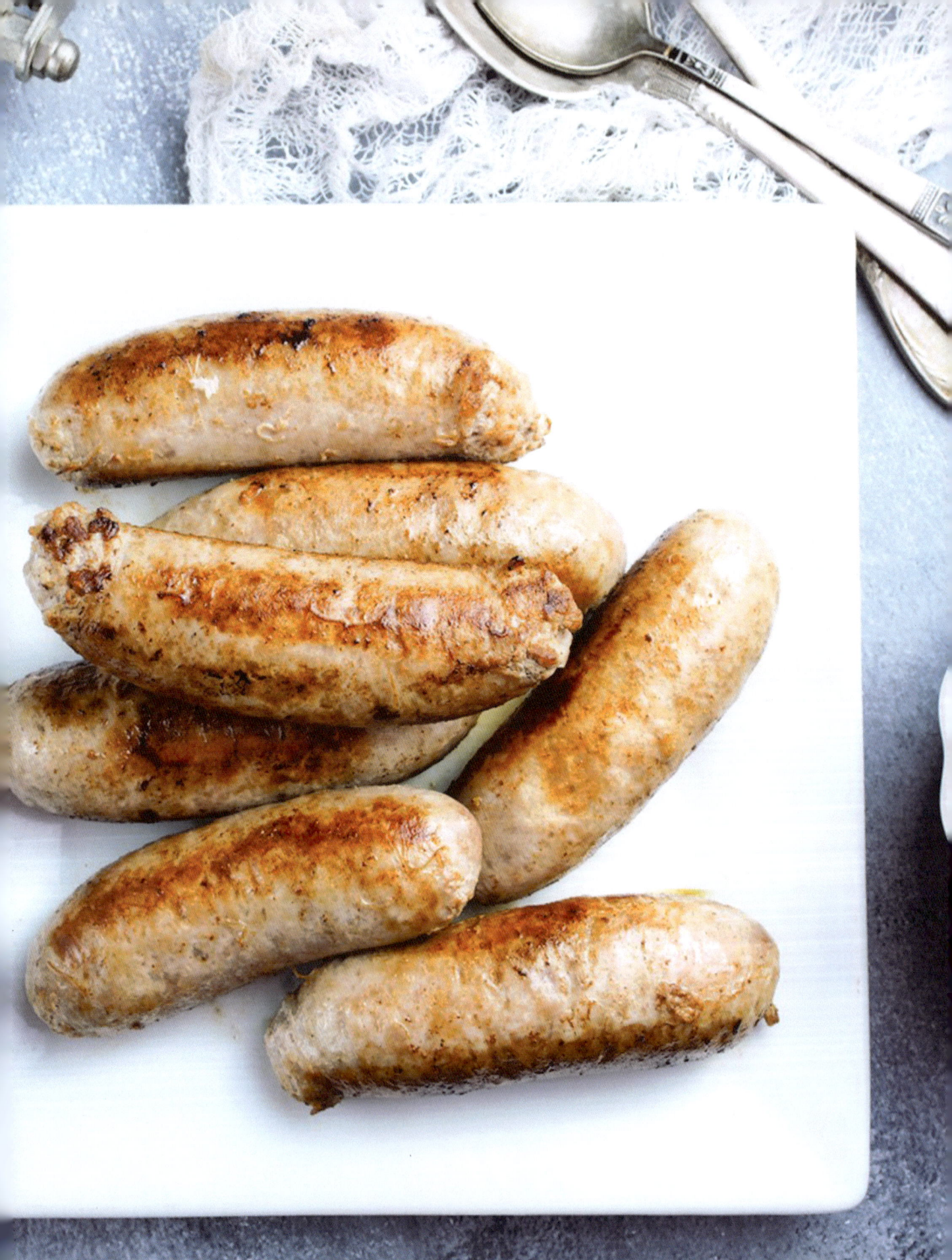

SAUSAGE, COURGETTE & TOMATO RISOTTO   Serves 4

INGREDIENTS:

- 7 sausages
- 2 tbsp coconut oil
- 1 cup Arborio rice
- 1 onion, diced
- 1 tbsp olive
- 14 cherry tomatoes, halved
- 2 garlic cloves, minced
- 1 cup tomato passata
- 1/2 tsp ground coriander
- 1 3/4 cups vegetable stock
- 2 courgettes, halved, sliced
- 1/3 cup parmesan, grated
- 1/4 cup yoghurt
- Pepper (to taste)
- Salt (to taste)

METHOD:

- Preheat the oven to 200°C. Place the sausages on an oven tray. Grill and cook for around 25 minutes or until cooked through and slightly golden. When done, slice into chunks. Add the cherry tomatoes and courgette on a separate oven tray and drizzle with the olive oil. Sprinkle with salt and pepper. Cook for around 10 minutes until tender.

- Meanwhile, heat the coconut oil in a pan and add the garlic and onion. Add the ground coriander and rice before gradually adding in the stock and passata a minute later. Bring to the boil then reduce to a simmer. Cover and cook for 20 minutes, making sure to stir occasionally.

- Once the rice is fully cooked, stir through the tomatoes, courgette, sausage and yoghurt and cook for a final 5 minutes. Taste and add more salt and pepper if necessary. Turn off the heat, serve up and garnish with the parmesan.

"Did you ever stop to taste a carrot? Not just eat it, but taste it?

You can't taste the beauty and energy of the earth in a Twinkie."

— ASTRID ALAUDA

HADDOCK WITH SWEET & SMOKY RED PEPPER STEW

Serves 2-4

INGREDIENTS:

- 4 haddock fillets
- 5 tbsp coconut oil
- 4 bell peppers, seeded, chopped
- 1 red onion, sliced
- 2 cups potatoes, cubed
- 3 garlic cloves, minced
- 4 cups vegetable stock
- 1 cup tomato sauce
- 1 cup tomatoes, diced
- 3 tbsp honey
- 2 tsp paprika
- 2 tbsp parsley, chopped
- Pepper (to taste)
- Salt (to taste)

METHOD:

- Preheat the oven to 180°C. Grease an oven tray with 1 tbsp of coconut oil. Lay the haddock fillets skin side down in the tray and add another tbsp of coconut oil on top. Sprinkle with salt. Bake for around 20 minutes until the fish is cooked but still moist.

- Heat the remaining coconut oil in a soup pot. Add the onion for 5 minutes until softened and then add the garlic, potatoes and bell peppers with some salt and pepper and cook for a further 10 minutes.

- Next, add in the tomatoes, tomato sauce, honey and stock. Bring to the boil and then reduce to a simmer. Cover and cook for 30 minutes.

- Finally, remove from the heat and stir through the parsley. Serve immediately.

SALSA VERDE STEAK SALAD — Serves 4

INGREDIENTS:

- 4 5oz steaks
- 2 shallots, diced
- 3 carrots, peeled, sliced
- 6 tbsp olive oil
- 2 tbsp coconut
- 6 cups spinach
- 30 cherry tomatoes
- 6 cups rocket
- 2 tbsp capers, chopped
- 6 tbsp parsley leaves, chopped
- 6 tbsp red wine vinegar
- Salt (to taste)

METHOD:

- Preheat the oven to 180°C. Salt the steaks. Place the carrots on an oven tray with 1 tbsp coconut oil and some salt. Toast in the oven for 10 minutes before adding the tomatoes for a further 10 minutes. Cook until the vegetables are softened and slightly golden.

- Combine the shallots and red wine together and let sit for at least 15 minutes. In a separate bowl, combine the olive oil, capers, parsley and some salt and pepper. Next, mix the shallots, but not the vinegar, into the oil-herb mix. Mix and then add in small amounts of the vinegar to taste.

- Meanwhile, heat a frying pan with the remaining coconut oil. Sear the steaks and cook to your desired level (2 minutes each side for rare, 5 minutes each side for well done). Once done, remove from the pan, and set aside.

- Plate the salad, slice the steak and then layer on top of the leaves. Top with the carrots and tomatoes and then drizzle with the salsa verde.

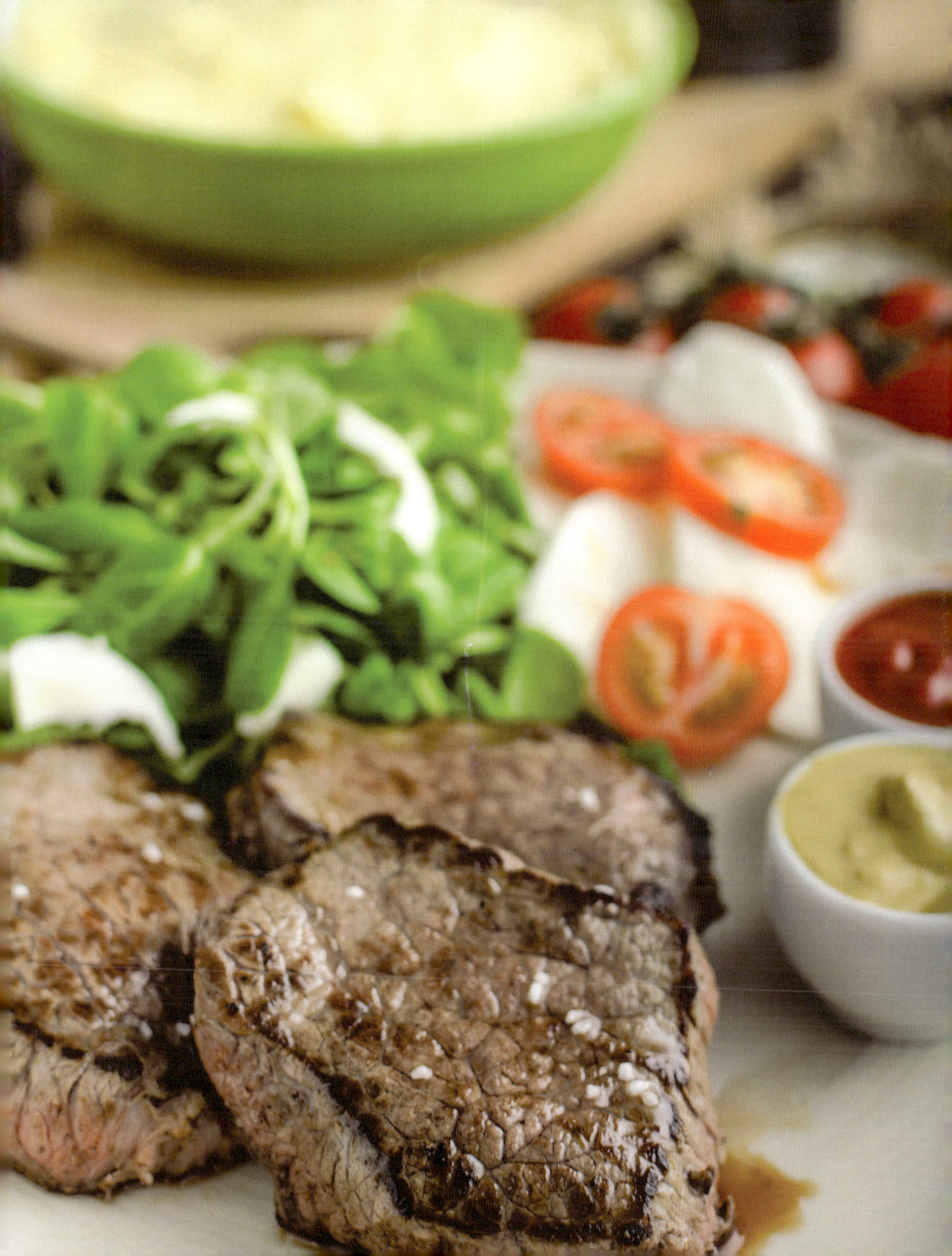

OLIVE & SUN-DRIED TOMATO STUFFED CHICKEN   Serves 2

INGREDIENTS:

- 2 chicken breasts
- 5 cups spinach
- 2 tbsp olive tapenade
- 1 onion, diced
- 1 tbsp olive
- 2 tsp dried basil
- 2 garlic cloves, minced
- 1 cup sun-dried tomatoes, finely chopped
- 3 tbsp butter
- 2 1/2 cups potatoes, quartered
- Pepper (to taste)
- Salt (to taste)

METHOD:

- Salt the chicken breasts and cut a pocket in the thickest part of them. Preheat the oven to 180°C. Mix the garlic, sun-dried tomatoes, basil and tapenade together. Stuff the mix in the chicken breasts before placing them in an ovenproof dish. Then, drizzle with the olive oil. Cook in the oven for around 25 minutes until cooked through.

- Meanwhile, add the potatoes and some salt to a pot of water and bring to the boil. Simmer for around 15 minutes until tender. When done, mash them thoroughly.

- Next, in a frying pan add the butter and onion. Fry for 5 minutes before adding a splash of water and the spinach. Cook until wilted and then mix into the mashed potato.

- Serve the chicken alongside the mashed potato.

AGRODOLCE-TOSSED SQUASH, SPROUTS & STEAK   Serves 2-4

INGREDIENTS:

- 1 butternut squash, peeled, seeded
- 4 5oz steaks
- 6 tbsp red wine vinegar
- 2 tbsp honey
- 5 tbsp coconut oil
- 4 tbsp olive oil
- 1 garlic clove, minced
- 1/2 red onion, sliced
- 5 cups Brussels sprouts, trimmed, halved
- 1 tbsp mint, chopped
- Salt (to taste)

METHOD:

- Preheat the oven to 200°C. Half the squash and then slice into half crescents. Rub with half the coconut oil and sprinkle in salt. Mix the sprouts with the remaining the coconut oil and some more salt. Place them all on an oven tray and cook for 30 minutes until golden.

- Meanwhile, mix the onion with the vinegar and leave to sit for at least 15 minutes.

- Next, heat a frying pan over a medium to high heat. Add in the remaining coconut oil and then fry the steak. I recommend cooking the steak to rare which takes about 2 minutes each side. Once done, remove from the heat, slice and set aside.

- Once the vegetables are cooked, mix them together with onion and vinegar mix. Serve with the steak.

PRAWNS WITH PATATAS BRAVAS & ROASTED MANGE TOUT   Serves 2

INGREDIENTS:

1 1/2 cups prawns, peeled
2 tbsp tomato puree
2 tsp paprika
4 tbsp olive oil
1 lemon, zested, juiced
1 tbsp honey
3/4 cup mange tout
2 large potatoes, diced

2 tbsp rice flour
1/2 cup vegetable stock.
1/4 cup butter
2 tbsp sun-dried tomato paste
2 garlic cloves, minced
1 onion, diced
Pepper (to taste)
Salt (to taste)

METHOD:

- Preheat the oven to 180°C. Place the potatoes on an oven tray with some salt and 1 tbsp olive oil. Cook for around 25 minutes until tender and golden. Place the mange tout on another oven tray and drizzle with 1 tbsp olive and sprinkle with some salt. Cook until tender (about 10 minutes).

- Meanwhile, heat a frying pan with the butter and some salt and cook the prawns and garlic for around 5 minutes. Once cooked, add in some of the lemon juice and zest to taste.

- In another pan, heat up the onions with the remaining olive oil and some salt. Cook for 5 minutes before adding in the tomato puree, tomato paste, paprika, honey and gradually pouring in the stock. Cook for another 5 minutes until the sauce thickens.

- Plate the prawns next to the mange tout and potatoes. Drizzle the potatoes with bravas sauce and the prawns with the lemon-butter sauce.

CHEESY CHICKEN, MUSHROOM & BROCCOLI PASTA   Serves 2

INGREDIENTS:

3 chicken breasts, diced
1 cup mushrooms, sliced
1 broccoli head, trimmed, chopped
2 cups rice penne
1 tbsp olive oil

3 tbsp butter
1/2 cup chicken stock
2 garlic cloves, minced
1/2 cup parmesan, grated
Salt (to taste)

METHOD:

- Salt the chicken. Boil two pots of salted water. Add the broccoli to one and simmer until it is tender but still has a slight bite to it. In the other pot, add the olive oil and cook the penne until it is tender but still has a slight bite to it.

- Meanwhile, heat a frying pan with the butter and add the chicken. Cook until the outside is no longer pink and then add the garlic and mushrooms, cooking for a further minute. Add the chicken stock, bring it to the boil and simmer until the chicken is cooked through, approximately 15-20 minutes. Turn off the heat.

- Next, add in the penne and broccoli to the chicken pan before stirring in the parmesan. Serve immediately.

CHICKEN THIGH, POTATO & VEG TRAY ROAST Serves 2

INGREDIENTS:

4 chicken thighs, skin on
1 tbsp white wine vinegar
1 tbsp olive oil
1 1/2 cups potatoes, halved
1 1/2 cup kale, torn
1 cup green beans, trimmed, halved

2 tbsp honey
1 large red onion, sliced into wedges
2 garlic cloves, minced
1 leek, chopped
Salt (to taste)

METHOD:

- Salt the chicken thighs. Preheat the oven to 200°C. Lay the leeks, onion, potatoes and green beans on an oven tray. Add the thighs on top and toss the whole tray with the olive oil, honey, garlic and some salt.

- Roast for around 30 minutes before adding the kale. Cook for a further 10 minutes until everything is cooked and the vegetables are tender.

- When done, serve up the food immediately. Drizzle in the vinegar to the oven tray and mix with the juices. Use this as a simple gravy.

SWEDISH-STYLE PORK MEATBALLS WITH COURGETTI   Serves 2

INGREDIENTS:

1 onion, diced
2 cups pork mince
3 tbsp butter
1 1/2 cups pork stock
1 cup goats double cream
1 tbsp honey
1 tbsp Worcestershire sauce

1 tsp Dijon mustard
1 tsp ground coriander
2 courgettes
1 tsp paprika
2 garlic cloves, minced
Pepper (to taste)
Salt (to taste)

METHOD:

- Preheat the oven to 200°C. Make the meatballs by combining the mince, paprika, garlic, onion powder, ground coriander and some salt and pepper in a bowl.

- Shape into meatballs and place on an oven tray grill. Cook for around 15 minutes until cooked through and slightly browned.

- Meanwhile, boil a pot of salted water then reduce to a simmer.

- Spiralize the courgette or thinly slice it into long spaghetti-like pieces if you don't have a spiralizer.

- Place in the boiling water for 2-5 minutes until tender.

- Next, heat a pan with the butter and then add in the stock, cream, mustard, Worcestershire sauce, honey and some salt and pepper.

- Bring to a gentle simmer and then add in the cooked meatballs. Cook for a few minutes before removing from the heat.

- Plate the courgetti and then top with the meatballs and sauce.

SPICY LAMB KOFTA KEBABS WITH YOGHURT DRESSING

Inspired by **EndoBoss® Alumni** - Jessica Le Gray from UK   Serves 2

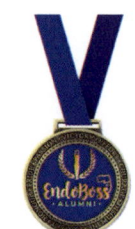

INGREDIENTS:

2 cups lamb mince
1 onion, finely diced
1 egg
3 rice cakes, crushed
1 bell pepper, chopped
1 chilli pepper, finely chopped
1 tsp cumin
1 tsp cinnamon
1 tbsp honey
1 tsp paprika

1 cup thick yoghurt
1 tbsp olive oil
1/4 lemon, juiced
1 tbsp white wine vinegar
1 tsp dill, chopped
4 garlic cloves, minced
1 tsp cayenne pepper
Pepper (to taste)
Salt (to taste)

METHOD:

- Soak 6 wooden skewers. Preheat the oven to 180°C.
- Combine the mince, onion, egg, rice cakes, cumin, cinnamon, paprika, half the minced garlic, cayenne pepper and some salt and pepper.
- Then form 6 kebabs on the wooden skewers. Place on an oven tray grill and cook for about 25 minutes, or until cooked through and golden on the outside.
- Meanwhile, make the yoghurt dressing. Combine the yoghurt, lemon juice, remaining minced garlic, olive oil, white wine vinegar, honey, dill and some salt.
- Serve together and dip the kebabs into the yoghurt dressing. You can also use tomato sauce or mayonnaise if you prefer.

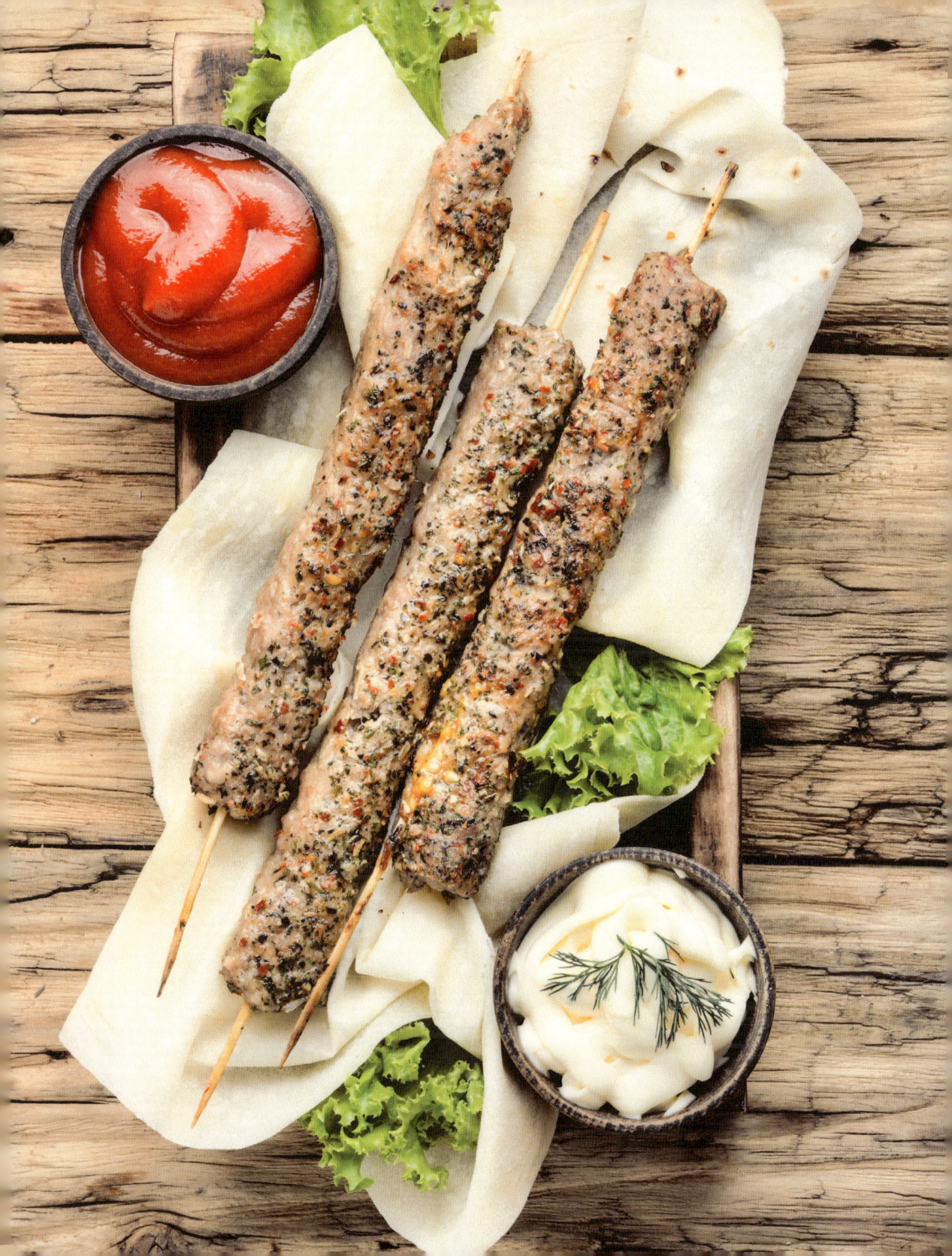

MANGO SALSA CHICKEN SALAD — Serves 2

INGREDIENTS:

- 2 chicken breasts
- 1/2 red chilli, seeded, finely chopped
- 2 tsp harissa paste
- 2 tbsp honey
- 1/2 lime, juiced
- 1 cup spinach
- 1 cup rocket leaves
- 1 tbsp coconut oil
- 1 cup lettuce
- 1 small red pepper, diced
- 2 tbsp coriander, chopped
- 1 half avocado
- 1/2 cucumber, diced
- 1 mango, peeled, pitted, diced
- 1/4 red onion, diced
- 1 cup of small tomatoes
- Salt (to taste)

METHOD:

- Salt the chicken. Preheat the oven to 200°C. In a bowl, mix the coconut oil, harissa paste, 1 tbsp honey and some salt. Put the chicken in an oven dish and spread with the harissa sauce.

- Cook for around 25 minutes until cooked through. When the chicken is done, cut into slices.

- Meanwhile, make the mango salsa by mixing the onion, mango, avocado, pepper, coriander, cucumber, chilli, lime juice, remaining honey and some salt together in a bowl.

- To serve up, plate the spinach and rocket leaves. Top with the mango salsa and then place the chicken on top.

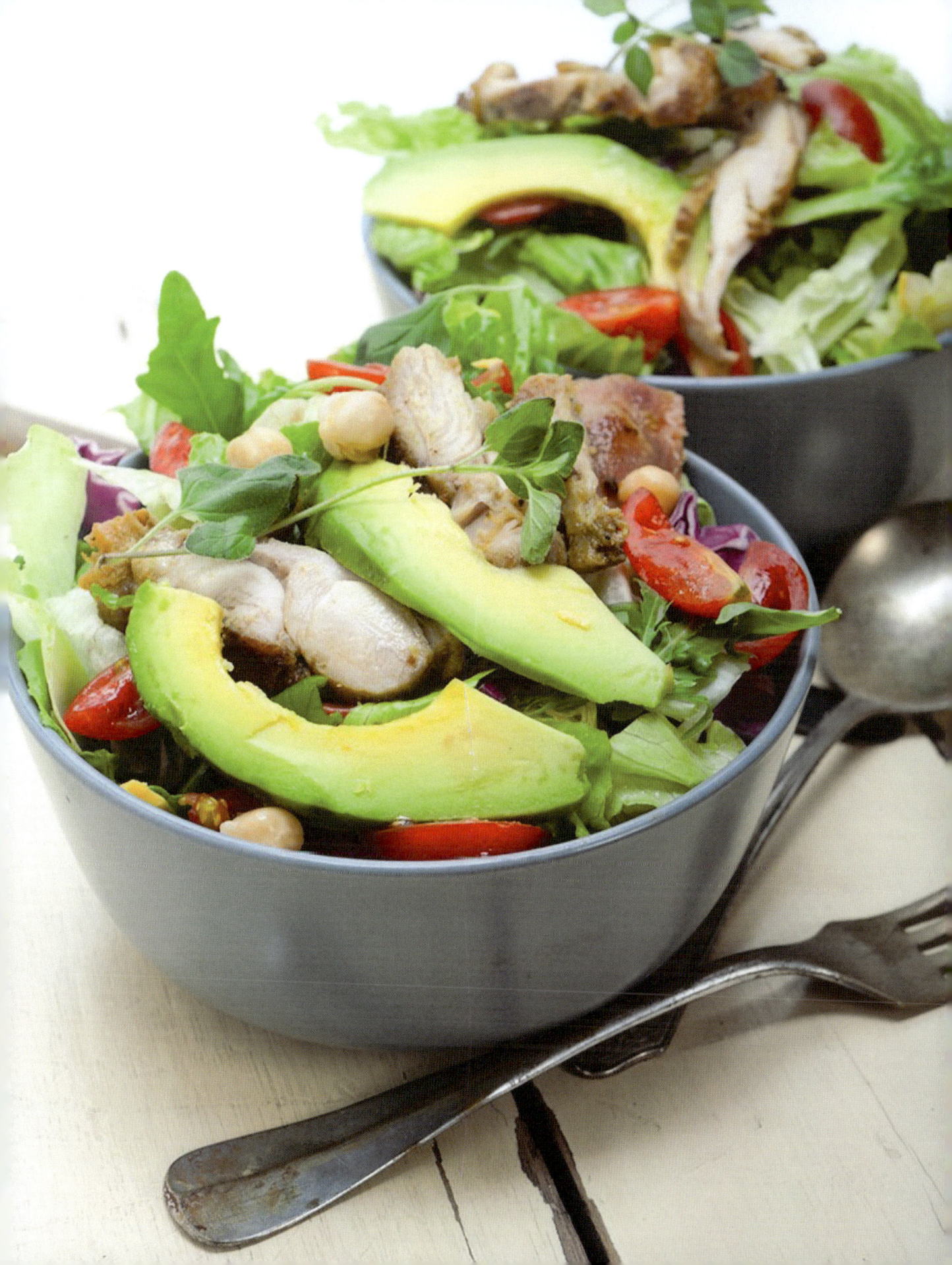

HADDOCK NOODLE PUTTANESCA

Serves 2-4

INGREDIENTS:

- 4 haddock fillets
- 1 onion, sliced
- 2 garlic cloves
- 2 tbsp olive oil
- 2 tbsp capers
- 1/4 cup olives, pitted
- 2 tbsp parsley, chopped
- 2 cups rice stick noodles
- 1/4 cup anchovy fillets, chopped
- 1 1/4 cups cherry tomatoes, chopped
- Salt (to taste)

METHOD:

- Preheat the oven to 180°C. Sprinkle the haddock fillets with some salt.

- To make the puttanesca, heat the oil in a pan and fry the onion for 5 minutes until slightly softened. Then, add in the garlic and cook for a further 5 minutes before adding in the tomatoes, olives, capers, anchovies and some salt and pepper.

- Once the mixture has been brought to a simmer, transfer to an ovenproof dish and nestle the haddock fillets in the puttanesca. Cook in the oven for around 15 minutes until the fish is cooked.

- Meanwhile, bring a pot of salted water to the boil and then add in the rice noodles. Cook them for about 3-5 minutes until just soft to bite. Drain and serve onto plates, spooning the puttanesca and haddock on top. Garnish with the parsley.

FRIED SEABASS & SQUASH PUREE   Serves 2

INGREDIENTS:

2 seabass fillets
2 red onions, cut into wedges
2 courgette, sliced
4 tbsp coconut oil
1/2 tsp cinnamon
2 tbsp honey

2 carrots, cut into batons
1/2 orange, zested, juiced
1/3 cup yoghurt
1 butternut squash, halved lengthways, seeded
Salt (to taste)

METHOD:

- Preheat the oven to 200°C. Season the seabass with salt. Put the squash halves on an oven tray, skin side down. Mix 2 tbsp coconut oil, the honey, orange juice and some salt in a bowl. Pour evenly over each half, adding any excess into the well in either half. Toast in the oven until soft (about 45 minutes).

- Place the courgettes, carrots and red onions on another oven tray with some salt and 1 tbsp coconut oil. Toast in the oven for around 20 minutes until softened and slightly golden.

- Meanwhile, fry the seabass in a frying pan with the remaining coconut oil. Cook the skin side first until crispy. Then, flip the fish and top the skin with the orange zest before frying for a few minutes.

- Once the squash is done, mash into a smooth puree. Make sure to include the coconut oil and honey juices in the puree. Mix in the cinnamon and add some more salt if desired.

- To serve, spoon the puree onto a plate and flatten. Place the seabass in the centre and then surround with the roasted vegetables.

BEEF STROGANOFF & CAULIFLOWER RICE   Serves 4

INGREDIENTS:

- 2 tbsp coconut oil
- 1 garlic clove, minced
- 2 tbsp butter
- 1 tsp Dijon mustard
- 1 large cauliflower head, trimmed, chopped
- 1/3 cup beef stock
- 2/3 cup creme fraiche
- 4 5oz beef steaks, sliced
- 3 cups mushrooms, sliced
- 4 tbsp parsley, chopped
- 1 onion, diced
- Salt (to taste)

METHOD:

- Salt the beef. Heat 1 tbsp coconut oil in a frying pan and tip in the onion with some salt and pepper. Cook for about 10 minutes until softened. Add in the garlic and cook for a further few minutes. Next, add in the butter and once beginning to foam, add the mushrooms to the pan. Continue to cook for 5 minutes before removing everything from the pan.

- Heat the remaining coconut oil in the pan and add the beef. Fry for about 3-5 minutes until browned. Return the vegetables to the pan and mix in the stock, creme fraiche and mustard. Cook for another 5 minutes.

- Meanwhile, place the cauliflower in a pot of salted water. Bring to the boil and cook for about 10 minutes until very soft. Drain and roughly mash. Stir in half the parsley. Plate the cauli rice with the stroganoff before garnishing with the remaining parsley.

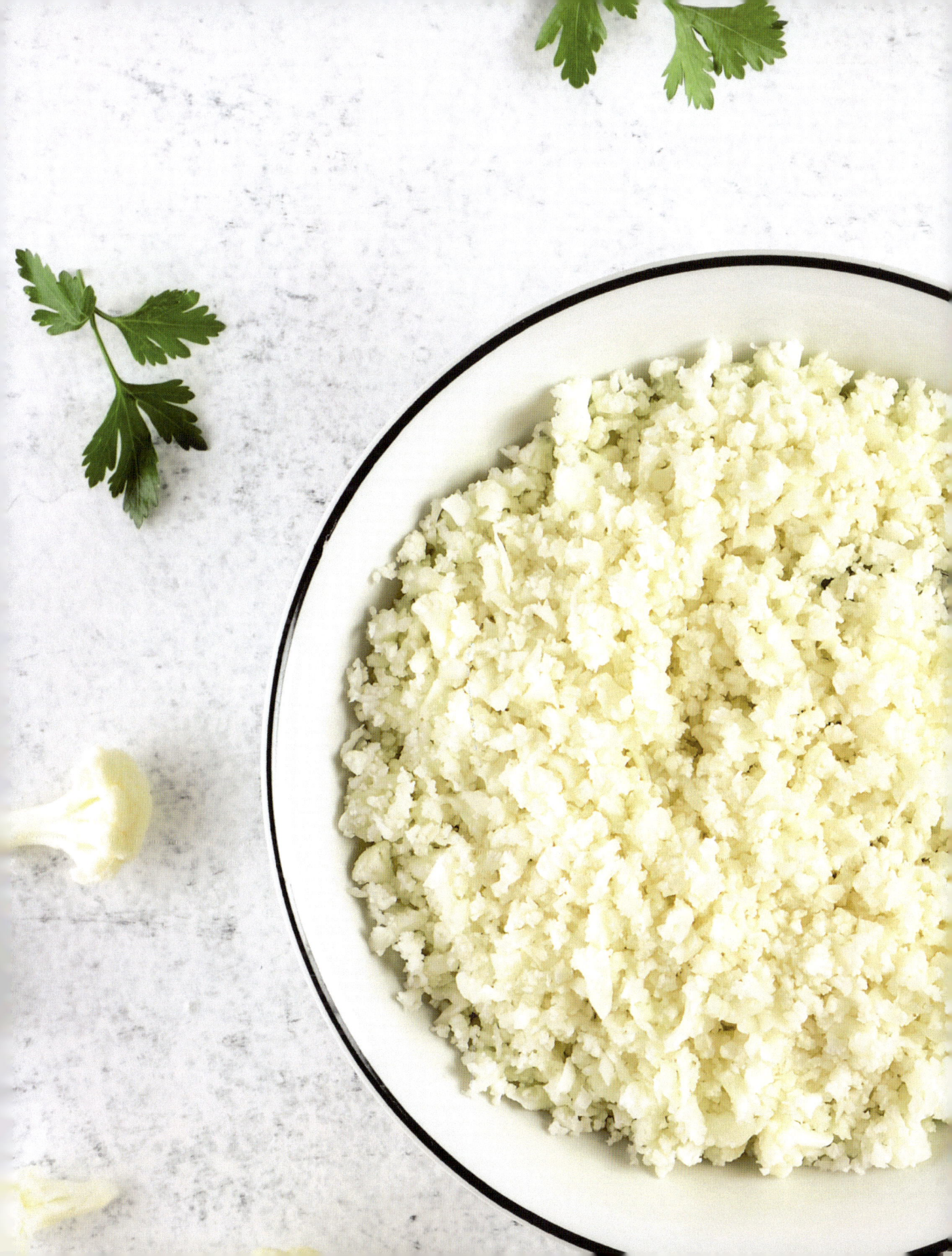

"*Our lives are not in the lap of the gods, but in the lap of our cooks.*"

– LIN YUTANG

SWEET CHILLI SALMON WITH DAUPHINOISE POTATOES Serves 2-4

INGREDIENTS:

- 4 salmon fillets
- 5 tbsp sweet chilli sauce (ensure it is great quality)
- 1 tbsp ginger, minced
- 2 tbsp olive oil
- 2 garlic cloves
- 4 large potatoes, finely sliced
- 1 cup double cream
- 3/4 cup milk
- 1/2 cup cheese, grated
- 1 tbsp Worcestershire sauce
- 3 cups tenderstem broccoli
- 2 spring onions, sliced
- Pepper (to taste)
- Salt (to taste)

METHOD:

- Sprinkle the salmon fillets with salt and pepper. Preheat the oven to 180°C. Combine the ginger, Worcestershire sauce, sweet chilli and some salt. Bring the cream, milk, garlic and some salt to a simmer in a large pan. Add the sliced potatoes and cook for around 5 minutes. Transfer the mix to an oven dish, discarding the garlic in the process. Sprinkle the grated cheese on top and bake for around 30 minutes until the potatoes are tender and slightly charred.

- Meanwhile, add the salmon fillets skin side down to an oven tray that has been greased with 1 tbsp of olive oil. Cook for 5 minutes and then pour in the sweet chilli sauce mixture. Cook for a further 5 minutes until the salmon is cooked.

- Then, place the broccoli on an oven tray with the remaining olive oil and some salt. Cook until tender and starting to crisp (about 15 minutes).

- Once it is all cooked, transfer to plates and serve immediately.

SPROUTS & LARDONS WITH JACKET POTATOES   Serves 2-4

INGREDIENTS:

4 cups Brussels sprouts, quartered

2 cups lardons

4 jacket potatoes

3 tbsp coconut oil

Salt (to taste)

METHOD:

- Preheat the oven to 180°C. Make sure the jacket potatoes are bone dry and then prick their skin with a fork. Rub all over with 2 tbsp coconut oil and sprinkle with salt. Then place on an oven tray and bake for around 60-90 minutes, or until the skin is crispy and golden, and the centre is soft.

- Meanwhile, heat a pan with the remaining coconut oil. Fry the lardons until crispy and then set aside. Toss in the sprouts with some salt and cook in the lardon fat until tender and slightly golden. Mix in the lardons and remove from the heat.

- Once the potatoes are done, slice open and spoon in the cooked sprout and lardon mix. Drizzle in the fat and juices from the pan and sprinkle with more salt if desired. Serve immediately.

SUPER SCRUMPTIOUS SOUPS

"You don't have to cook fancy or complicated masterpieces — just good food from fresh ingredients."

– JULIA CHILD

ROMAN EGG DROP SOUP Serves 4-6

INGREDIENTS:

8 cups chicken stock
6 eggs
1 tbsp olive oil
2 onions, diced
4 tbsp parmesan, grated

2 tbsp parsley, chopped
Pepper (to taste)
Salt (to taste)

METHOD:

- Whisk together the eggs with the parmesan, parsley and some salt and pepper. Heat a soup pot and add the olive oil.

- When the oil is heated, add the onions and cook until tender.

- Next, add the stock and bring to a simmer.

- Pour the egg mixture into the stock in a thin stream, whilst gently whisking the soup. Be careful not to over mix which will break up the eggs into tiny bits; you are wanting them in long rags.

- Once all the mixture is added, turn off the heat. Taste the soup and add more salt if necessary.

- Serve up and garnish with more grated parmesan if desired.

WENDY'S SIMPLE & DELICIOUS PEA SOUP   Serves 2-4

INGREDIENTS:

8 cups peas (or full bag of frozen peas)

2 onions, sliced

2 1/2 cups vegetable stock (about 2 stock cubes dissolved in 2 1/2 cups of water)

Salt (to taste)

METHOD:

- Heat a soup pot over a medium heat and add the butter. Once melted, add in the onions and reduce the heat.

- Soften the onions for about 10 minutes, adding water if they start to brown.

- When done, add the peas with enough stock to cover them. Crank up the hob to a high heat and simmer for 15 minutes.

- After this, blend the mixture. Add more stock if you need a thinner consistency. Taste and add more salt if needed.

- To lift the flavour of the soup even more, add a dash of apple cider or white wine vinegar and mix well.

You can use this recipe template to make a simple soup from any vegetable. Just simply switch out the peas and replace with an equal amount of the other vegetable.

TOMATO SOUP   Serves 4

INGREDIENTS:

3 cups fresh tomatoes, chopped
2 tbsp honey
2 garlic cloves, sliced
2 bay leaves, halved
2 tsp tomato puree
2 tbsp olive oil
2 tbsp basil, chopped

1 carrot, diced
1 celery rib, diced
1 onion, sliced
4 cups vegetable stock
Pepper (to taste)
Salt (to taste)

METHOD:

- Heat the oil in a soup pot and add in the carrot, onion, celery, garlic and some salt. Cook for around 10 minutes until they become soft and lose some colour.

- Next, add in the tomato puree and the chopped tomatoes along with the honey, bay leaves, and some pepper. Mix everything together and then cover and allow to stew for a further 10 minutes. Stir occassionally.

- Then, pour in the stock and bring to the boil. Turn down the heat to bring it to a simmer and cover again, allowing to cook for about 25 minutes.

- Finally, once cooked, remove from the heat, discard the bay leaves and stir through the basil. Blend up the soup and then taste, adjusting with extra salt, pepper and honey if necessary. Add more tomato puree if you wish for the colour to be a deeper red.

- Garnish with additional basil leaves if desired.

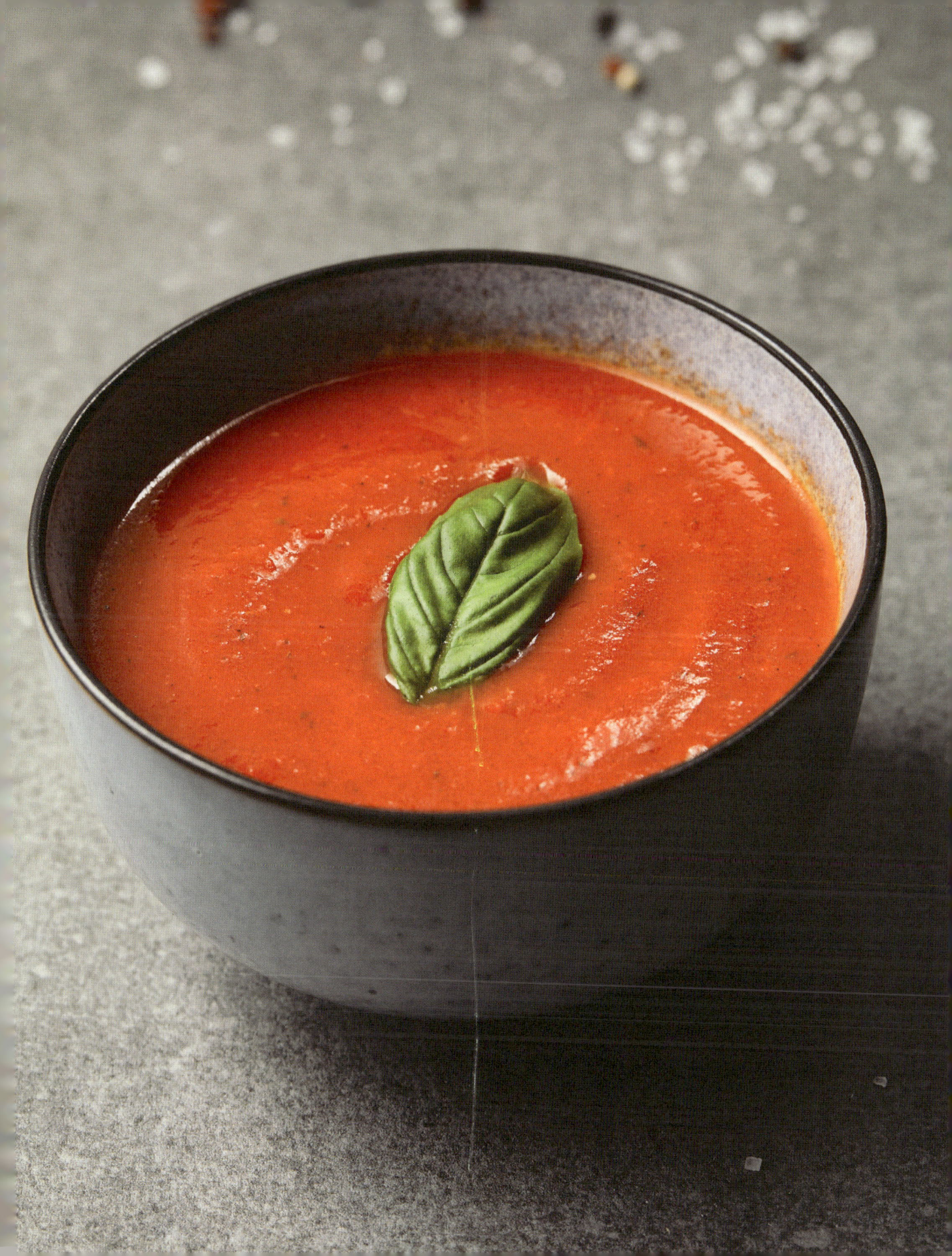

VEGETABLE MEDLEY SOUP — Serves 4

INGREDIENTS:

1 onion, sliced
4 celery ribs, diced
4 carrots, diced
2 bell peppers, seeds and core removed, sliced
2 leeks, sliced
2 courgettes, sliced
3 large potatoes, diced
2 bay leaves
4 tbsp olive oil
3 garlic cloves, sliced
3 cups vegetable stock
Pepper (to taste)
Salt (to taste)

METHOD:

- Heat the oil in a soup pot and add in the carrots, celery ribs, onion and some salt. Cook for 5 minutes until softened and fragrant.

- Next, stir in the garlic, potatoes, bay leaves, leeks, peppers and courgettes. Cook for another 5 minutes.

- Then pour in the stock and some pepper. Bring the mixture to the boil and then simmer for around 15 minutes until all the vegetables have softened.

- Remove from the heat, discard the bay leaves and then blend up the soup until smooth. Add more stock if a thinner consistency is needed.

- Taste and add more salt and pepper if needed. Serve hot.

CHICKEN NOODLE SOUP   Serves 2-4

INGREDIENTS:

1 1/2 cups cooked chicken, torn
4 cups chicken stock
1 tsp fresh ginger, chopped
1 small onion, diced
1 garlic clove
1 tbsp coconut oil

1/2 cup rice noodles
3 chestnut mushrooms, thinly sliced
2 spring onions, diagonally sliced
2 tbsp parsley, chopped
4 tbsp sweetcorn
Salt (to taste)

METHOD:

- Heat the stock in a pan with the garlic, ginger, onion, coconut oil and some salt.
- Simmer for a few minutes before adding the chicken, noodles, sweetcorn, mushrooms and spring onions.
- Continue to simmer until the noodles are soft. Then, serve and garnish with the parsley.

> *"He was a bold man that first ate an oyster."*
>
> — JONATHAN SWIFT

CREAMY SWEETCORN, LEEK & POTATO SOUP   Serves 4

INGREDIENTS:

4 cups sweetcorn

1 1/2 cups baby potatoes, diced

2 cups chicken stock

1 1/2 cups leeks, chopped

2 onions, sliced

1/2 cup butter

Salt (to taste)

METHOD:

- Heat a pot of water to boiling and add in the potatoes and lots of salt. Cook for 20 minutes then run with cold water, drain and set aside.

- Meanwhile, heat the butter and some salt over a medium heat in a soup pot. Once melted, add the onions and cook until softened. If they start to brown, add a splash of water.

- Once done, add in the leeks and cook for 5 minutes before adding in the sweetcorn and cooking for a further 5 minutes.

- Next, add enough stock to cover all the ingredients in the pan. Simmer for around 10 minutes.

- Then blend up the soup thoroughly before adding the potatoes into the pot and cooking for a further 5 minutes. Once cooked, serve up and enjoy!

TUSCAN KALE SOUP — Serves 4-6

INGREDIENTS:

- 4 cups kale, chopped
- 4 cups chicken stock
- 1 onion, diced,
- 2 tbsp olive oil
- 1/2 cup pancetta, diced
- 2 celery ribs, diced
- 3 carrots, diced
- 2 bay leaves
- 2 garlic cloves, minced
- 2 cups chopped tomatoes
- 1 tsp dried oregano
- 1 tsp dried basil
- 1/2 lemon, juiced
- Pepper (to taste)
- Salt (to taste)

METHOD:

- Heat up a stock pot over a medium heat and add 1 tbsp olive oil, and some salt and pepper. Once the oil is heated, add the pancetta until it begins to brown.

- At that point, add the carrots, onion, celery and bay leaves. When the veg is tender add in another tbsp of olive oil and pour in the tomatoes, garlic, oregano and basil.

- Let the ingredients simmer for 10 minutes and then add in the kale and enough stock to cover it all. Cook for another 15-20 minutes until the kale is tender and stir through the lemon juice. Taste and add more salt if necessary.

- Before serving, remove the bay leaves. For extra flavour, drizzle in some more extra virgin olive oil.

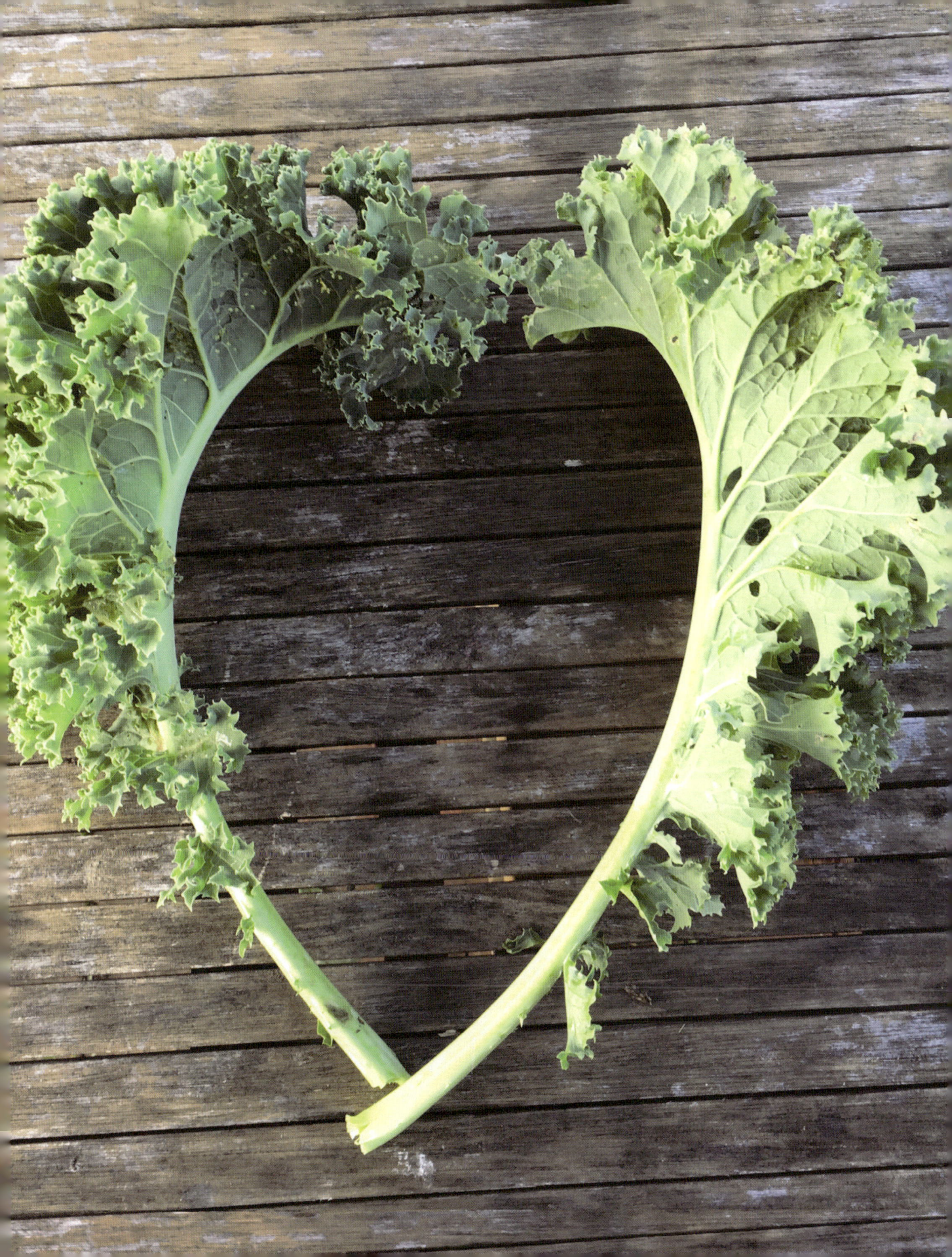

SWEET POTATO & COCONUT SOUP   Serves 4

INGREDIENTS:

1 onion, sliced

1 tbsp coconut oil

2 tbsp Thai green curry paste

4 cups vegetable stock

1 cup coconut cream

2 tbsp coriander, chopped

2 tbsp desiccated coconut

5 1/2 cups sweet potato, cubed

Salt (to taste)

METHOD:

- Melt the coconut oil in a soup pot and add the sweet potato and some salt. Cook until slightly golden. Next, add the onion and cook until softened and then add the curry paste for 1 minute.

- Then, add the stock and simmer for 20 minutes. Once done, remove from the heat and add in the coconut cream and coriander.

- Taste and add more salt if needed. Blend into a creamy liquid.

- Heat a separate pan and add the desiccated coconut. Cook it until golden and toasted.

- Serve up the soup and garnish with the toasted coconut.

SPINACH & DILL SOUP WITH FETA   Serves 4-6

INGREDIENTS:

6 stalks of fresh parsley
2 garlic cloves, sliced
2 bay leaves
1 carrot, diced
1 celery rib, diced
3 onions, diced
3 cups vegetable stock
5 cups spinach
2 tbsp olive oil
2 medium potatoes, diced
1/2 cup dill sprigs, chopped
1 tbsp red wine vinegar
1 1/2 cups feta, crumbled
Pepper (to taste)
Salt (to taste)

METHOD:

- Heat the oil in a soup pot and add in the carrot, celery, onion and some salt.
- After 5 minutes, add the garlic, parsley and bay leaves, ensuring to regularly stir them. Cook until fragrant.
- Next, add in the vegetable stock and the potatoes. Bring to the boil, simmer for 15 minutes and then add in the spinach, red vinegar, half the dill and some pepper. Stir until the spinach wilts.
- When ready, discard the bay leaves. Then, blend up and taste. Adjust with salt and pepper, and more stock if necessary.
- Serve hot with the feta mixed through. Garnish with the remaining dill.

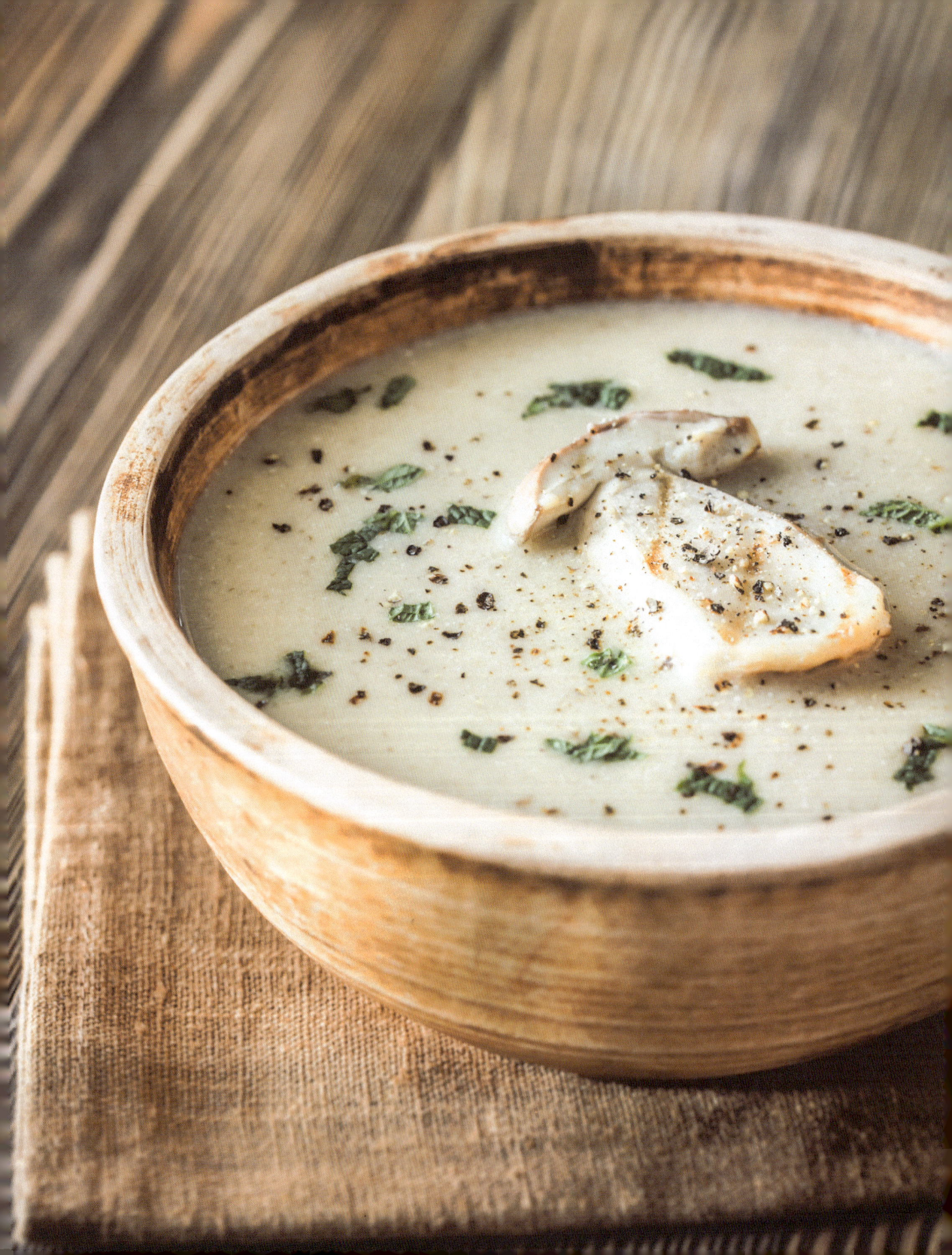

CREAMY MUSHROOM SOUP — Serves 6

INGREDIENTS:

- 5 tbsp butter
- 2 onions, sliced
- 6 tbsp rice flour
- 8 cups mushrooms
- 2 tbsp white vinegar
- 4 tsp parsley, chopped
- 2 beef stock cubes
- 1 cup double cream
- 4 cups chicken stock
- 4 garlic cloves, minced
- Pepper (to taste)
- Salt (to taste)

METHOD:

- Heat the butter in a soup pot and add in the onion until softened before adding the garlic and cooking for a further minute.

- Add in the mushrooms and cook for 5 minutes, stirring occasionally, and then pour in the white wine vinegar and cook for another minute.

- Next, sift in the flour and mix well before cooking for 2 minutes. Add in the chicken stock with some salt and pepper and bring the mixture to a boil.

- Once boiled, reduce to a simmer and crumble in the beef stock cubes before covering and allowing to cook for around 15 minutes. Continue to stir occasionally.

- Once done, turn off the heat, pour in the cream and stir through with the parsley.

- Taste and adjust the seasoning with salt and pepper if necessary. Serve immediately.

"High-tech tomatoes. Mysterious milk. Super-squash. Are we supposed to eat this stuff? Or is it going to eat us?"

– ANNITA MANNING

ROASTED AUBERGINE SOUP WITH HARISSA   Serves 4

INGREDIENTS:

2 cups chopped tomatoes

2 tbsp olive oil

2 tbsp coconut oil

3 tbsp harissa paste

4 aubergines, cubed

1 onion, diced

2 cups vegetable stock

2 tbsp coriander, chopped

Salt (to taste)

METHOD:

- Preheat the oven to 200°C. Place the aubergine on an oven tray and spread with some salt and the coconut oil.

- Cook in the oven for about 15-20 minutes until browned and softened. You may need to mix them around during this time.

- Next, heat the oil in a soup pot. Add the onion, cook until soft and then add the harissa paste and cook for 2 minutes.

- Then, add the aubergines and cook for a further few minutes before adding in the stock, some salt and the tomatoes. Bring to the boil and simmer for 15 minutes.

- Once ready, blend into a smooth liquid and stir through the coriander. Taste and adjust with salt if necessary.

POTATO-LEEK SOUP WITH CRISPY PANCETTA Serves 6-8

INGREDIENTS:

3 cups of leeks, only the white parts, diced
1/4 cup butter
3 cups potato, diced
1 onion, diced
4 cups vegetable stock
1/2 cup milk
1/2 cup cream
1 1/2 cups pancetta, diced
Pepper (to taste)
Salt (to taste)

METHOD:

- Melt the butter in a soup pot and then add in the potatoes, leeks, onion and some salt and pepper. Mix well for a minute and then place the lid on the pot.

- Next, place the lid on the pot and cook over a gentle heat for around 10 minutes until the vegetables soften. Then, pour in 3 cups of the stock and bring to the boil. Simmer the vegetables for around 15 minutes until cooked.

- Meanwhile, heat up a frying pan and cook the pancetta until golden and crispy. Set aside when done.

- Turn off the heat when ready and blend into a smooth liquid. Taste and adjust with salt and pepper if necessary. Finally, add in the milk and cream.

- Gently reheat the soup and add more of the final cup of vegetable stock to thin the consistency if desired. Serve hot and generously top with the crispy pancetta.

BUTTERNUT SQUASH & GREEN CURRY SOUP WITH FRIED SHALLOTS & CORIANDER   Serves 4

INGREDIENTS:

3 tbsp coconut oil
1 onion, sliced
2 garlic cloves, minced
2 cups vegetable stock
4 cups butternut squash, peeled, seeded, cubed
1 can thick coconut milk
1/2 lime, juiced

1 tsp ginger, minced
2 shallots, diced
2 tbsp Thai green curry paste
1/3 cup coriander, chopped
Pepper (to taste)
Salt (to taste)

METHOD:

- Heat 2 tbsp of the coconut oil in a soup pot and add in the garlic and onion.
- Cook for around 5 minutes until softened and then add in the ginger, curry paste and some salt and pepper. Cook for a further few minutes and then add in the butternut squash.
- After 5 minutes add in the stock. Bring to the boil and then simmer until the squash is tender (around 20 minutes).
- Meanwhile, add the remaining coconut oil to a frying pan. Heat over a medium heat and then fry the shallots with some salt until crispy.
- When the squash is tender, turn off the heat and pour in the coconut milk and lime juice. Blend thoroughly and then taste and adjust with salt and pepper if necessary.
- Stir through the coriander or reserve as a garnish when serving up.

CARROT, TURNIP & CORIANDER SOUP   Serves 4

INGREDIENTS:

3 cups carrots, chopped

3 turnips, chopped

2 tbsp olive oil

1 tsp ground coriander

1 onion, sliced

4 cups vegetable stock

1/2 cup goats or coconut yoghurt

2 tbsp goats or coconut milk

1/3 cup coriander, chopped

Pepper (to taste)

Salt (to taste)

METHOD:

- Heat the oil in a soup pot and cook the onion for around 5 minutes until softened. Stir in the ground coriander and cook for 1 minute.

- Then add in the carrots, turnips, the stock and some salt and pepper.

- Bring the mixture to the boil and then reduce to a simmer for 25 minutes making sure to cover with the lid.

- Cook until the carrots and turnips are tender.

- When ready, blend up the mixture into a smooth liquid. Taste and adjust the seasoning if necessary.

- Mix the yoghurt with the milk to thin it. Drizzle on top of the soup and add the chopped coriander on top to garnish the soup.

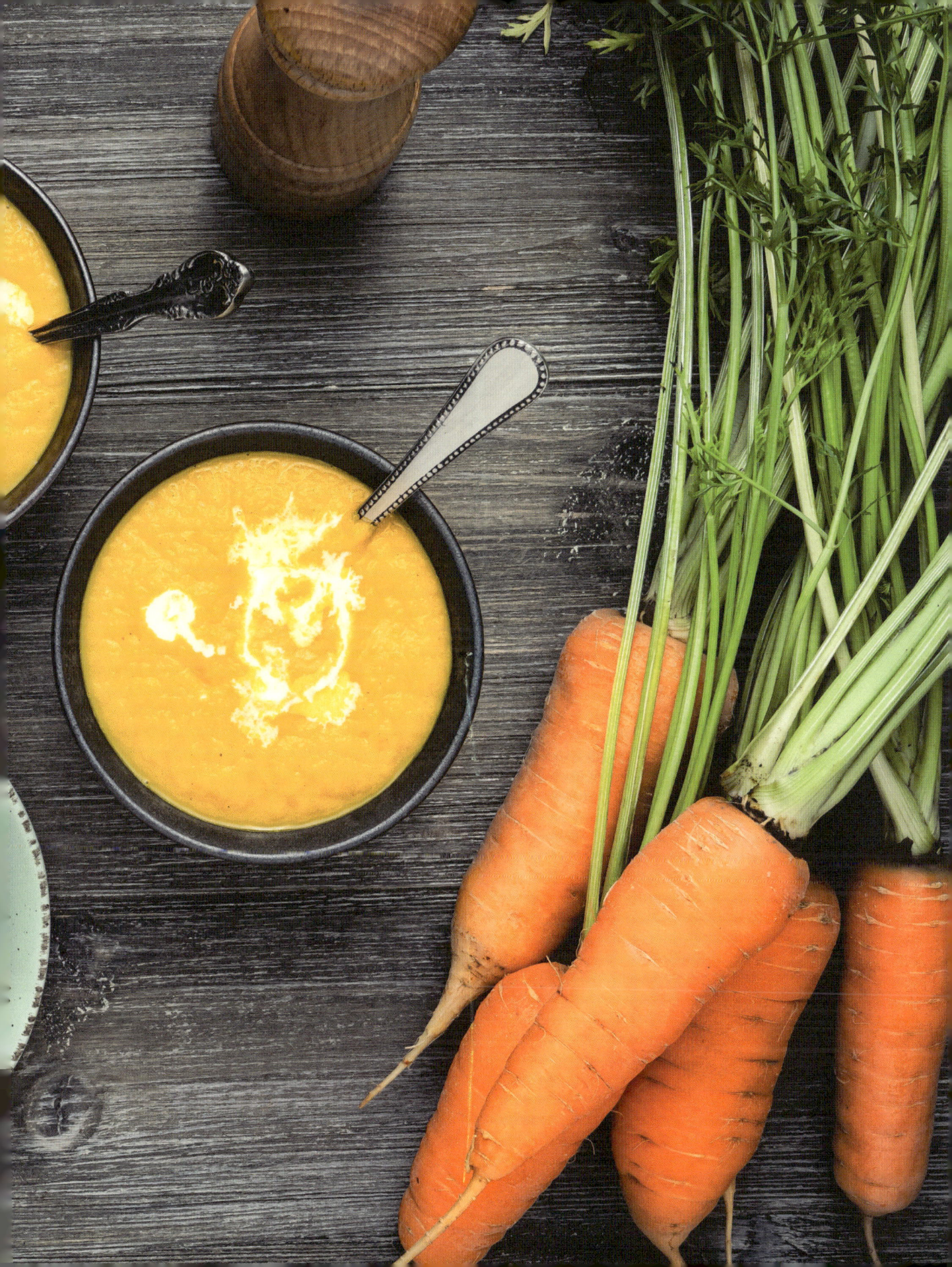

CHILLED CUCUMBER & YOGHURT SOUP

Serves 4

INGREDIENTS:

1 1/2 cups yoghurt
2 large cucumbers, seeded, chopped
1 shallot, diced
3 tbsp olive oil
1/2 lemon, juiced
1 garlic clove

1/4 cup parlsey, chopped
2 tbsp tarragon, chopped
1/3 cup dill, chopped
Pepper (to taste)
Salt (to taste)

METHOD:

- Combine all the ingredients in a blender and blitz together until a smooth liquid forms. Season with salt and pepper.

- Cover the soup and refrigerate for at least 8 hours.

- When ready to serve, taste and adjust with more seasoning if necessary. Garnish with chopped cucumber and some olive oil.

> *"If more of us valued food and cheer and song above hoarded gold, it would be a merrier world."*
>
> — J.R.R TOLKIEN

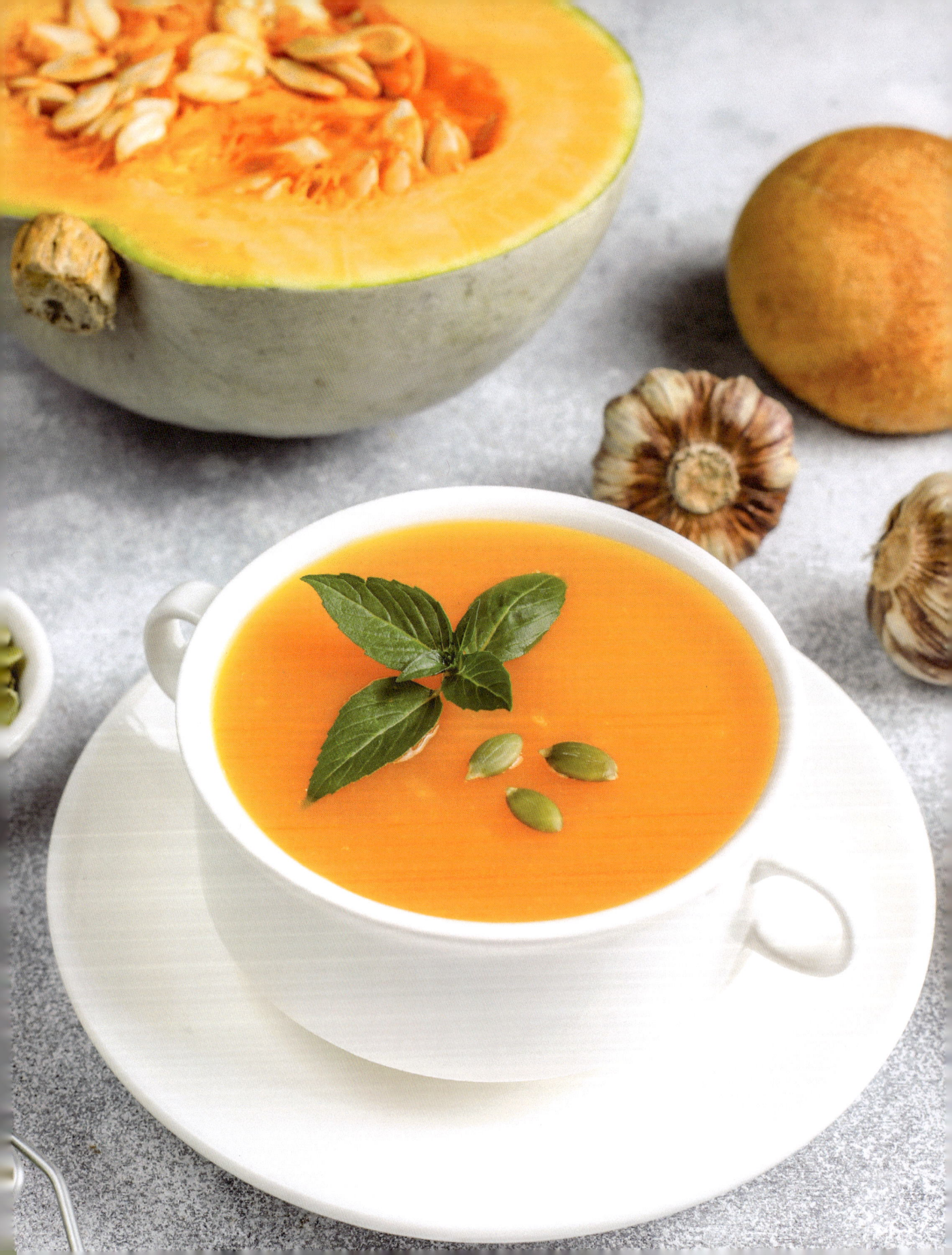

SPICED PUMPKIN SOUP — Serves 4-6

INGREDIENTS:

1 medium pumpkin, seeded, diced
1 onion, sliced
3 tbsp olive oil
2 tsp ground coriander
2 tsp cumin powder
3 1/2 cups vegetable stock
1/3 cup double cream
2 tbsp ginger, minced
3 garlic cloves, minced
Pepper (to taste)
Salt (to taste)

METHOD:

- Preheat the oven to 180°C. Place the diced pumpkin, with the skin still on, an oven tray and coat with 2 tbsp olive oil, 1 tsp coriander, 1 tsp cumin and some salt. Cook for around 30-45 minutes until very tender.

- Meanwhile, heat the remaining oil in a soup pot and cook the onion with some salt for 5 minutes until soft. Next, add the garlic, ginger, and remaining coriander and cumin. Cook for a few more minutes before pouring in the stock. Bring to the boil and then reduce to a simmer.

- Once the pumpkin is ready, remove the skin and then add into the pot with the cream. Turn off the heat and blend the mixture into a smooth liquid. Taste and adjust with more salt and pepper if necessary. Serve hot.

RICH GREEN SOUP — Serves 4-6

INGREDIENTS:

- 1 tbsp honey
- 1 broccoli head, trimmed, chopped
- 1 cauliflower head, trimmed, chopped
- 3 garlic cloves, sliced
- 8 cups spinach
- 2 bay leaves
- 1 tbsp olive oil
- 2 tbsp coconut oil
- 3 tbsp butter
- 1 tsp apple cider vinegar
- 2 carrots, diced
- 2 onions, sliced
- 4 1/2 cups chicken stock
- Pepper (to taste)
- Salt (to taste)

METHOD:

- Heat the coconut oil in a soup pot and add in the carrots for a few minutes to soften. Then put in the sliced onions until softened. After this, add the garlic and cook for a few more minutes until aromatic. Season with lots of salt.

- Next, add in the butter, stock, broccoli, cauliflower and bay leaves. Mix well and then cover and simmer for 15 minutes until the vegetables are very soft. Add in the spinach and cover for a further few minutes.

- Then, add in the honey, vinegar, olive oil and some pepper. Discard the bay leaves. Turn off the heat and blend into a smooth liquid.

- Taste and adjust the seasoning with salt and pepper if necessary. Serve immediately.

MULLIGATAWNY SOUP   Serves 4-6

INGREDIENTS:

4 cups chicken stock

1/4 cup white rice

1 carrot, diced

1 onion, diced

2 celery ribs, diced

4 tbsp butter

2 bay leaves

1/2 apple, cored, chopped

1 1/2 tbsp rice flour

2 tsp curry powder

1 chicken breast, diced

1/2 cup double cream

Pepper (to taste)

Salt (to taste)

METHOD:

- Heat the butter in a soup pot and add in the carrot, onion and celery with some salt. Cook until softened and then add in the flour, bay leaves and curry powder and cook for 5 mintues. Next, add in the stock, bring to the boil and then reduce to simmer for 10 minutes.

- Finally, add in the apple, chicken and rice and cook for 20-30 minutes, ensuring to cook the chicken thoroughly. When done, turn off the heat and stir through the cream. Serve hot.

"Eating good food is my favourite thing in the world. Nothing is more blissful."

- JUSTINE LARBALESTIER

ROASTED CAULIFLOWER SOUP   Serves 2-4

INGREDIENTS:

1 large head cauliflower, chopped
2 tbsp coconut oil
3 tbsp butter
1 rib celery, diced
2 onions, diced
1/4 lemon, juiced

2 garlic cloves, minced
4 cups vegetable stock
1/4 tsp cloves, ground
2 tbsp parsley, chopped
Pepper (to taste)
Salt (to taste)

METHOD:

- Preheat the oven to 200°C. Spread the coconut oil over the cauliflower. Place in an oven tray and sprinkle with salt. Toast until tender and slightly golden (about 20-30 minutes).

- Meanwhile, in a soup pot heat the butter and add in the onion and celery. Cook for around 5 minutes until softened. Then add in the garlic and some salt. After about a minute, pour in the stock. Add in the roasted cauliflower and bring the mixture to the boil, then reduce to a simmer and cook for 20 minutes with some occasional stirring.

- When the mixture is cooked, remove from the heat and add in the cloves, lemon juice and some pepper. Then, blend into a smooth liquid. Taste and adjust with salt and pepper if necessary. Serve up and garnish with the chopped parsley.

THE GREEN MACHINE SOUP   Serves 4

INGREDIENTS:

- 2 heads of broccoli, main stem removed, chopped
- 2 garlic cloves, minced
- 1 large potato, diced
- 1 onion, sliced
- 3 tbsp coconut oil
- 4 cups vegetable stock
- 2 tbsp parsley, chopped
- 1 leek, sliced
- 1 1/2 cups kale, torn
- 1 1/2 cups spinach
- Pepper (to taste)
- Salt (to taste)

METHOD:

- Heat the oil in a soup pot and add the onion and leek. Cook for 5-10 minutes until softened. Add in the potato, broccoli, parsley, garlic and some salt and pepper. Cook for a further 5 minutes before adding in the kale and stock. Bring the stock to the boil and then reduce to a simmer and place the lid on.

- Cook for around 25 minutes until the vegetables have softened. Then, add in the spinach. Cook for a final 5 minutes before removing the pot from the heat. Blend the mixture into a smooth liquid.

- Taste and adjust with salt and pepper if necessary. Serve hot.

PERFECTLY HEALTHY PUDDINGS

*"Life is uncertain.
So eat dessert first."*

—ERNESTINE ULMER

FLOURLESS BEETROOT BROWNIES

Serves 6-8

INGREDIENTS:

- 3 eggs
- 3/4 cup cooked beetroot, chopped
- 1/4 cup unsweetened cocoa powder
- 3/4 cup caster sugar
- 4 tbsp butter
- 2 teaspoons vanilla extract
- 2 1/2 cups dark chocolate
- Salt (to taste)

METHOD:

- Preheat the oven to 180°C. Blend or mash up the beetroot.

- In a bowl beat the butter and sugar together vigorously until fluffy. Then, add the eggs one at a time, beating with each addition. Next, add the vanilla, cocoa powder and some salt.

- Finally, melt the chocolate. Fold the melted chocolate and beetroot and mix until the batter is smooth and glossy.

- Pour the mixture into a greased baking tray and roughly flatten with a spoon. Put the tray in the oven and cook for around 15-25 minutes. Be careful not to over bake the brownies, the centre shouldn't jiggle when shaken but the batter should still be soft.

- When ready, remove from the oven and allow to cool for 10 minutes.

- Serve hot or place in the fridge to serve later when they will have more of a bite.

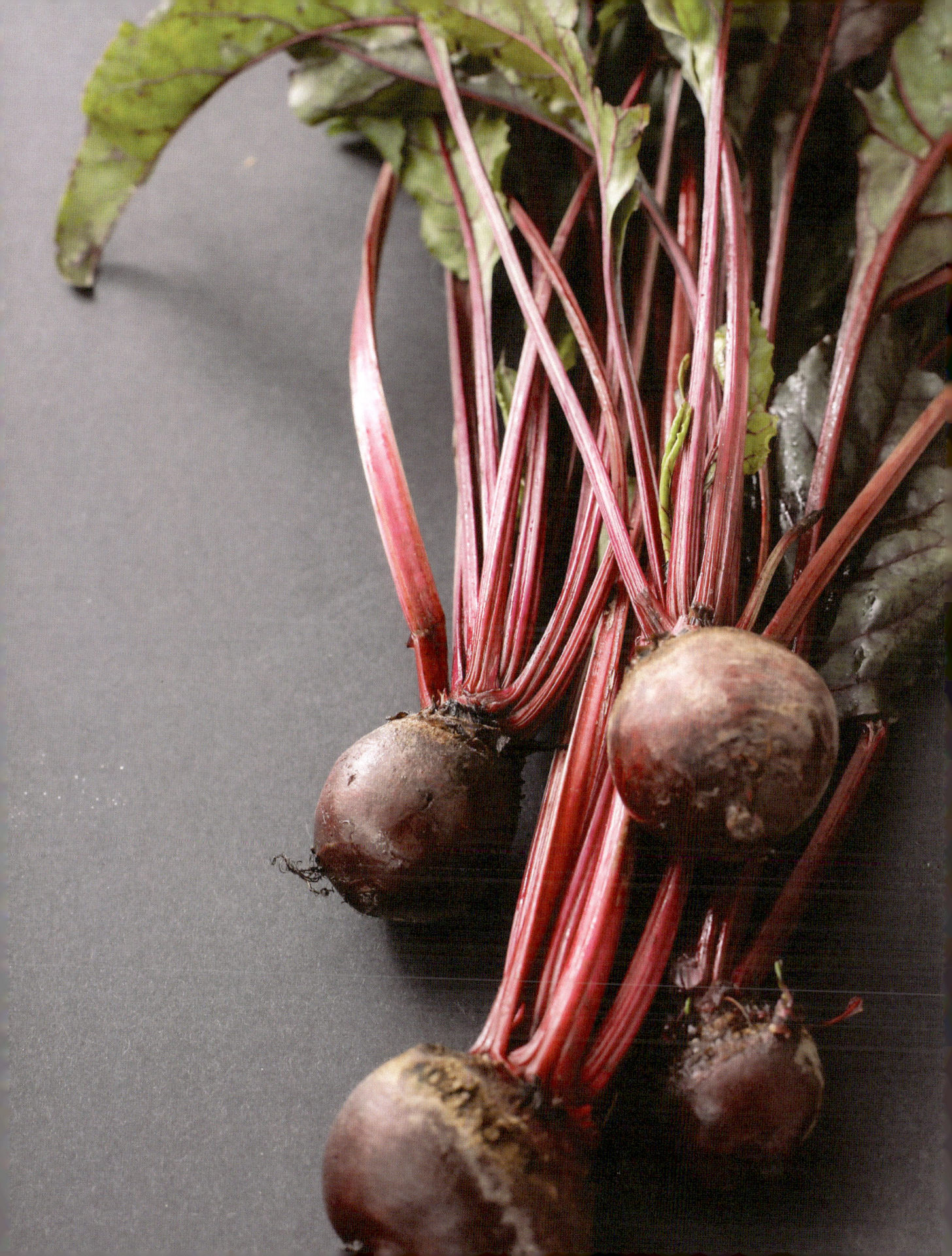

MELT IN THE MOUTH MAPLE MARSHMALLOWS

Serves 8

INGREDIENTS:

1 cup maple syrup
1 1/2 cups white sugar
7 tsp gelatin powder
1 tbsp vanilla extract
1 tbsp icing sugar
1 cup water
Salt (to taste)

METHOD:

- Mix the gelatin and half the water together. Set aside.

- Next, combine the remaining water with the sugar, syrup and some salt together in a pan. Gently heat until the sugar dissolves. Then, increase the heat and cook the mixture without stirring.

- After a few minutes spoon a small bit of the mixture into a bowl of ice cold water. If you are able to form a soft ball with the mixture then it is ready. If not, cook for a little longer and test again.

- Once ready, turn off the heat and gradually pour into the gelatin bowl, ensuring to whisk whilst doing so.

- When all of it has been poured from the pan, vigorously whisk for 3-5 minutes until thick and fluffy. Add the vanilla extract in the final minute of mixing.

- The mixture should be cool enough to touch. Spread it out on a flat ceramic dish and dust with the icing sugar. Getting your hands wet may help stop the marshmallow mix from sticking to your fingers.

- Set aside in a cool area for a few hours before slicing into squares.

CACAO & CAROB YOGHURT   Serves 4

INGREDIENTS:

3 cups yoghurt
1 tbsp carob
6 tbsp cocoa nibs
1/4 tsp vanilla extract
1/4 cup honey

1/2 cup dark chocolate, grated
Salt (to taste)

METHOD:

- Grind the cocoa nibs into a fine powder. Mix together in a bowl with the carob, honey, vanilla extract and some salt.
- Once done, serve up the yoghurt and top with cocoa mix.
- Garnish with the grated chocolate.

> "The proof of the pudding is the eating."
>
> — MIGUEL DE CERVANTES

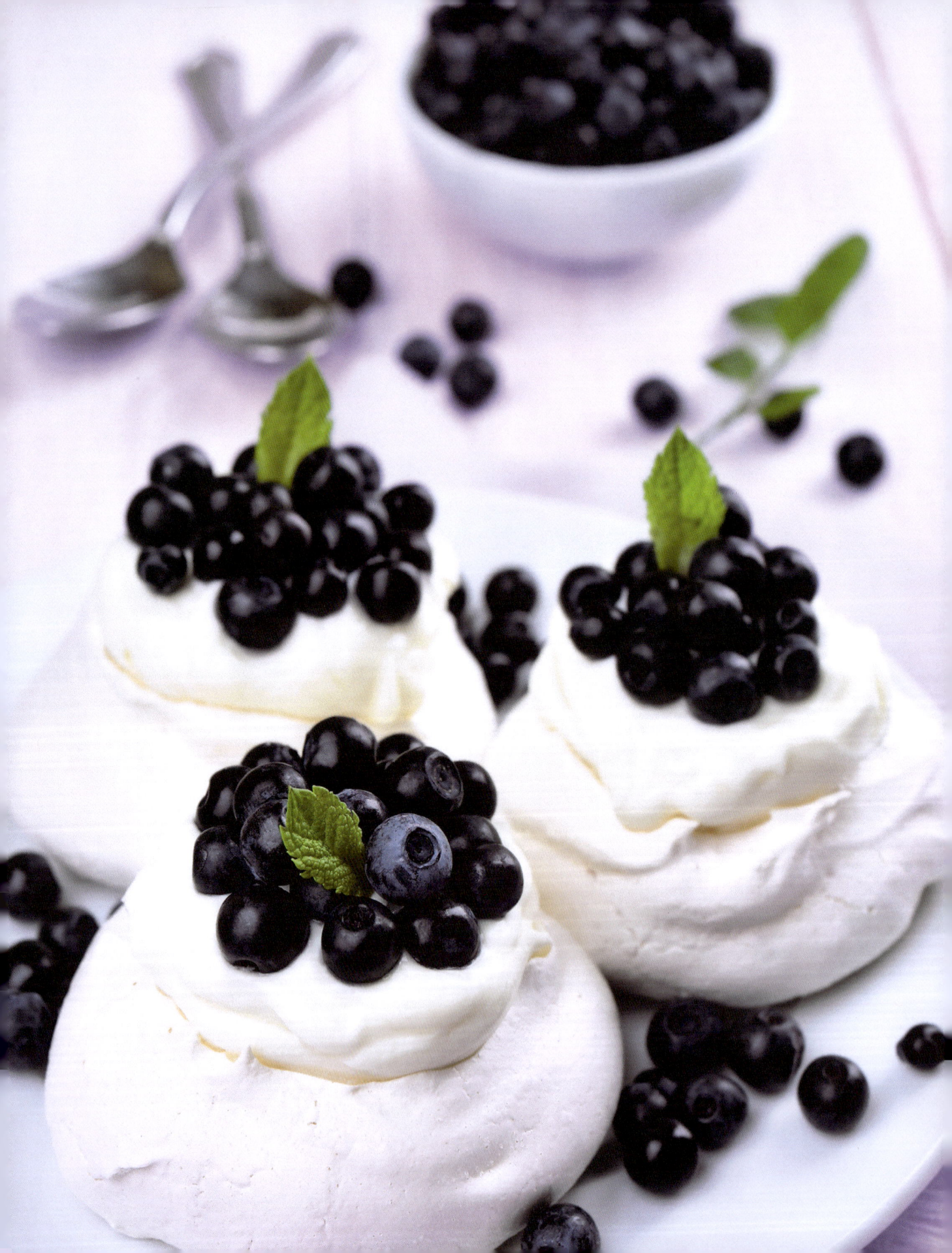

MAGNIFICENT MERINGUE CAKES   Serves 8

INGREDIENTS:

4 egg whites

1/2 cup caster sugar

1 cup icing sugar

1 cup of blueberries (optional)

METHOD:

- Preheat the oven to 100°C. Whisk the egg whites in a bowl until it is fluffy and stiff peaks form.

- Next, add the caster sugar, a spoonful at a time, and continue to whisk so the sugar mixes thoroughly into the egg whites. Adding the sugar slowly ensures that the meringues rise properly later. (Be careful not to over whisk; the mixture will look thick and glossy when ready).

- Repeat this step with the icing sugar but mix with a wooden spoon and sift in with a sieve instead.

- Now, dollop the mixture into round balls on a lined baking tray, making sure to leave space between each one.

- Cook for between 60-90 minutes until the meringues are crisp and a golden cream colour. Leave to cool before serving.

- Either serve as they are or consider serving with cream, yoghurt or ice cream dolloped on top and then finish off with blueberries.

PERFECT PEACH-MILK ICE CREAM FLOAT   Serves 4

INGREDIENTS:

2 cups peaches, destoned, diced

4 cups milk

1/4 tsp vanilla extract

4 cups coconut ice-cream

4 tbsp honey

Salt (to taste)

METHOD:

- Blend the honey, peaches, vanilla extract, milk and 2 cups of ice cream together with some salt.
- Once smooth, pour into glasses and top with the remaining ice cream.

Why not try to make your own ice-cream using the ice-cream recipe from later on in the recipe book?

"When it's raining pudding, hold up your bowl."

- SANDRA GALLAS

COCONUT RICE PUDDING — Serves 2-4

INGREDIENTS:

1/4 cup sugar
2 cups of milk
1/2 cup Arborio rice
1 can of thick coconut milk
1/2 cup desiccated coconut

Salt (to taste)

METHOD:

- Add the rice, milk, sugar, 2 cups of water and some salt to pan over a medium heat.

- Bring to the boil and then stir regularly for around 15-20 minutes until the rice is tender and sits in creamy sauce.

- Next, add in the coconut milk and simmer for a further 5-10 minutes until the rice has tenderised further and the sauce thickened.

- Meanwhile, toast the coconut in a separate pan, stirring regularly to avoid it burning.

- Once the coconut is golden, spoon it into the rice pudding.

- Mix well, and then serve up hot. Sprinkle with more toasted coconut to garnish if you would like!

BEE-EGG-NOG   Serves 4

INGREDIENTS:

4 egg yolks
Pinch cinnamon
Pinch ground nutmeg
2 tbsp bee pollen
1 tsp vanilla extract

2 cloves
1/2 cup double cream
2 cups milk
5 tbsp honey
Salt (to taste)

METHOD:

- Beat the yolks together and then add the honey, bee pollen and some salt. In a separate pan, heat the milk with the cinnamon and cloves.

- Once it starts to steam, turn off the heat. Be careful not to boil it as this will curdle the mix.

- Next, gradually pour the yolk mix into milk mix, making sure to stir consistently.

- Then stir in the vanilla extract, double cream and some more salt if needed.

- When serving, pour into glasses and sprinkle with the nutmeg.

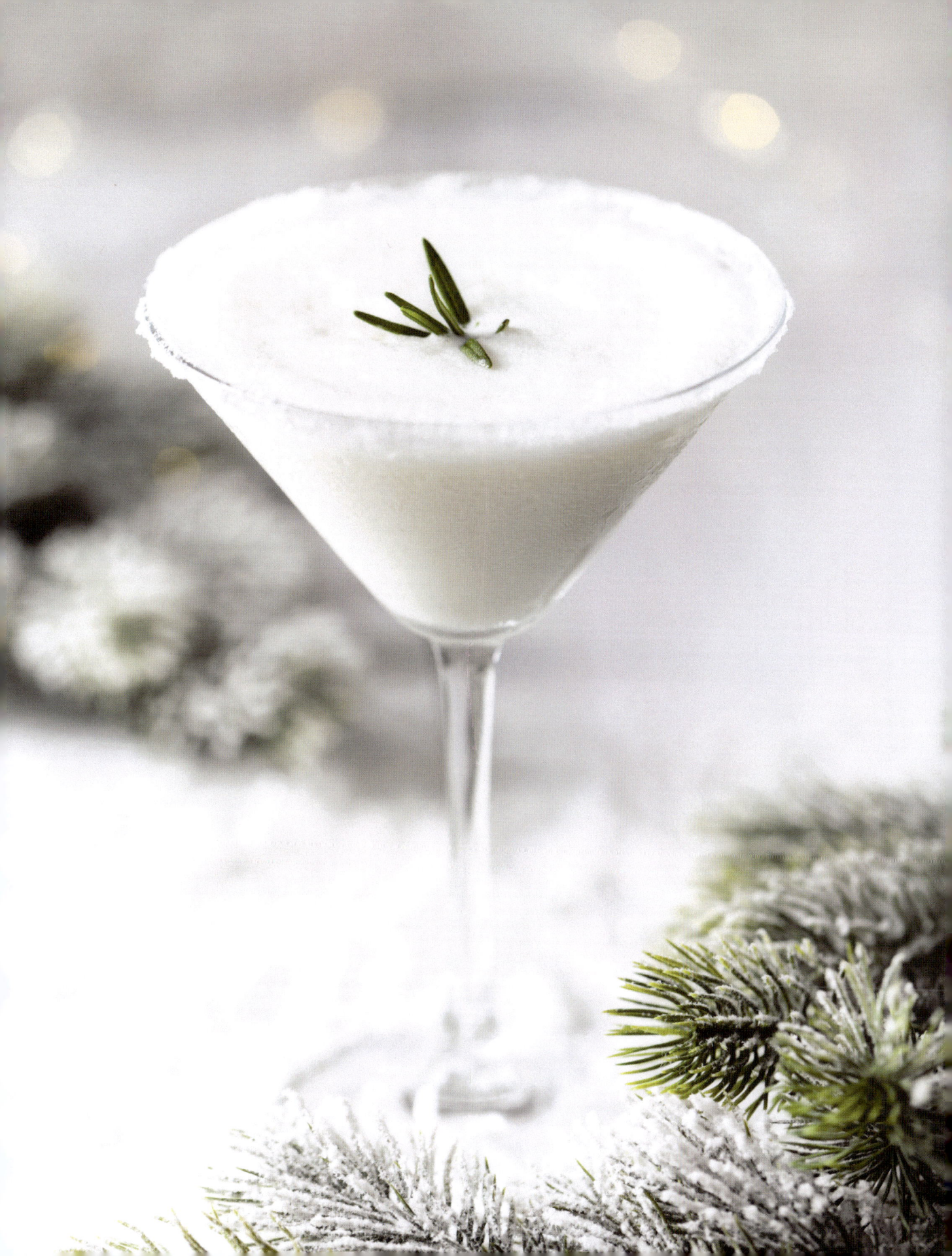

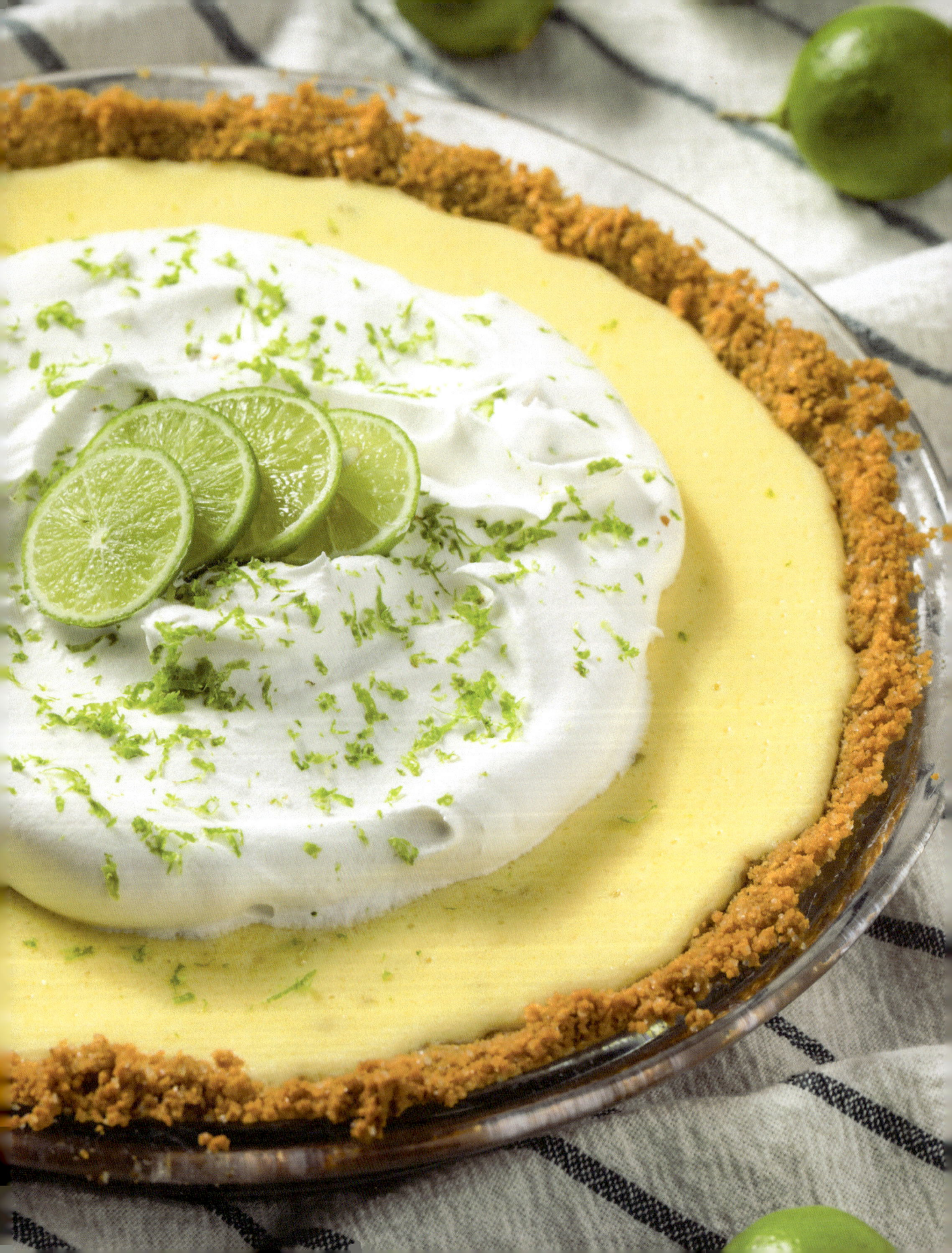

KEY LIME PIE   Serves 8-12

INGREDIENTS:

- 2 cups gluten-free oatcakes, crushed
- 1 cup butter
- 1 1/3 cups condensed milk
- 3 egg yolks
- 4 limes, zested, juiced
- 3 tbsp honey
- 1 1/4 cup double cream
- 2 tbsp icing sugar
- Salt (to taste)

METHOD:

- Preheat the oven to 160°C. Finely crush the oatcakes, melt the butter and then mix them together in a bowl with the honey and some salt.

- Once combined, spread the biscuit mix across the inside of a loose based tart tin (or a flat based dish if you don't have one). Making sure to evenly coat the sides of the tin or dish with the biscuit mix.

- Compact and flatten with a spoon and then bake in the oven for 10 minutes. Allow to cool for a while when done.

- Meanwhile, whisk the egg yolks for one minute before adding the condensed milk and whisking for a further few minutes.

- Finally, add the juice from the four limes and some zest (to taste). Whisk until fully combined.

- After the base has cooled, transfer the filling into the biscuit base and bake for 15 minutes. Next, allow to cool and then refrigerate for at least 3 hours.

- Before serving, whip the double cream and the icing sugar together until stiff peaks form. Dollop on top of the filling, garnish with some lime zest and lime slices.

- Finally, slice up and enjoy!

ENDOBOSS® BANOFFEE PIE Serves 6-8

INGREDIENTS:

1 1/2 cups gluten-free oatcakes
3/4 cup butter
1 1/3 cups condensed milk
1 tsp vanilla extract
1/3 cup muscovado sugar

1 1/4 cup double cream
2 bananas
2 tbsp honey
Salt (to taste)

METHOD:

- To make the biscuit base, finely crush the oatcakes and melt 1/2 cup butter. Mix together with the honey and some salt. Once combined, spread the biscuit mix across the inside of a loose-based tart tin making sure to equally coat the sides. Compact and flatten with a spoon and then place the tart tin in the fridge for at least 45 minutes.

- Meanwhile, start to make the caramel filling by heating the sugar and remaining butter in a pan over a low heat. Once combined, add the condensed milk. Whilst continuously stirring, bring the mixture to the boil and then keep cooking for 2-3 minutes until it turns a dark gold colour. Be careful not to burn the mixture or cook it too long.

- Remove from the heat when ready and mix in the vanilla extract and some salt. Pour in to the biscuit base and roughly flatten before refrigerating again for at least 15 minutes.

- Next, peel the bananas and then slice into discs. Whip the cream to stiff peaks being careful not to over-whip it. When the pie has cooled, layer the banana neatly on top of the caramel and then dollop the whipped cream on top of the banana layer.

- Slice up and enjoy!

COCO-CHOC FINGER BARS   Serves 2-4

INGREDIENTS:

3 tbsp coconut oil
1/4 cup cocoa butter
1/2 cup cocoa powder
5 tbsp honey
1 tsp vanilla extract

2 tbsp dessicated coconut
Salt (to taste)

METHOD:

- Melt the coconut oil and then combine with the cocoa powder, vanilla extract, honey, dessicated coconut and some salt.
- Mix well and then chill in thin chocolate molds or in rectangular dishes.
- Refridgerate for a few hours until solid. Enjoy!

"Life's a pudding full of plums."

— W.S. GILBERT

CANDIED EGG YOLKS — Serves 4

INGREDIENTS:

2/3 cup water

12 egg yolks

1 cup caster sugar

2 cup icing sugar

Salt (to taste)

METHOD:

- Add the sugar and water together in a pan and gently heat until boiling. Make sure to regularly stir.

- Simmer the mixture until a thick syrup forms and then remove from the heat.

- Meanwhile, whisk the egg yolks. When the syrup is ready, pour the yolks and some salt into it.

- Place the pan back on a gentle heat and stir continuously for a few minutes until the yolks begin to solidify. As this happens, the mixture will start to pull away from the sides of the pan.

- Remove from the heat and transfer to a flat tray to cool. Once cooled, sieve some extra icing sugar on top of the mixture.

- Finally, roll bits of the mixture into balls and cover with more icing sugar.

- Place the candied eggs yolks on a plate and refrigerate for at least 1 hour. Then serve and enjoy!

Serve as they are, place in small paper cases or add to ice cream.

GOOEY RICE PUFF SQUARES   Serves 8-10

INGREDIENTS:

9 cups rice puffs
3/4 cup butter
1/2 tsp vanilla extract
12 cups marshmallows (ensure good quality)
Salt (to taste)

METHOD:

- In a large pot, melt the butter with some salt. Add in the marshmallows and continue cooking until melted.
- Remove from the heat and stir in the vanilla extract and rice puffs.
- Once thoroughly mixed, transfer to a lined tray. Gently spread it with a spoon to fit the tray and very lightly press the mixture flat.
- Leave to set in the fridge for at least 1 hour before slicing into squares.

> "We are living in a world today where lemonade is made from artificial flavors and furniture polish is made from real lemons."
>
> – ALFRED E. NEWMAN

CREAMY CUSTARD — Serves 4-6

INGREDIENTS:

4 egg yolks
1 tsp vanilla extract
3 tsp gelatin powder
1/2 cup sugar
3 cups milk

1 cup double cream
Salt (to taste)

METHOD:

- Add the gelatin powder to 1/2 cup milk, mix and then set aside. Put the remaining milk in a pan with the cream and gently heat to just before boiling.
- Meanwhile, mix the yolks, sugar, vanilla and some salt together.
- When the heated milk mixture is ready, mix in the gelatin-milk.
- Then slowly mix together the milk mixture with the yolk mix.
- Transfer the mixture back into the pan and gently heat, making sure to stir regularly until the custard thickens. Ensure not to cook too long as lumps will form.
- Serve hot or cold and enjoy!

"Strength is the capacity to break a chocolate bar into four pieces with your bare hands – and then eat just <u>one</u> of the pieces."

– JUDITH VIORST

STRAWBERRY CHEESECAKE   Serves 8-12

INGREDIENTS:

- 3 cups gluten-free oatcakes, crushed
- 1 cup butter
- 1 cup double cream
- 1 cup icing sugar
- 3 tbsp honey
- 3 eggs, lightly beaten
- 2 1/2 cups full fat cream cheese
- 2 tsp vanilla extract
- 1 cup strawberries, sliced (to decorate)
- Salt (to taste)

METHOD:

- To make the biscuit base, finely crush the oatcakes, melt the butter and then mix together with the honey and some salt. Once combined, spread the biscuit mix across the bottom of a loose-based tart tin (or a flat based dish if you don't have one). Compact and flatten with a spoon and then refrigerate for about an hour until firm.

- Meanwhile, whisk the double cream until soft peaks begin to form. In a separate bowl mix the soft cheese, icing sugar, beaten eggs, vanilla extract and some salt until smooth and fully combined. Then, mixing the double cream. The mixture should be stiff enough to be able to stand on its own. If it can't, whisk for longer.

- Next, spoon the topping onto the biscuit base, ensuring there are no air bubbles.

- Smooth the top and place in the fridge for about 12 hours to set.

- When ready, decorate with the strawberries, slice up and enjoy!

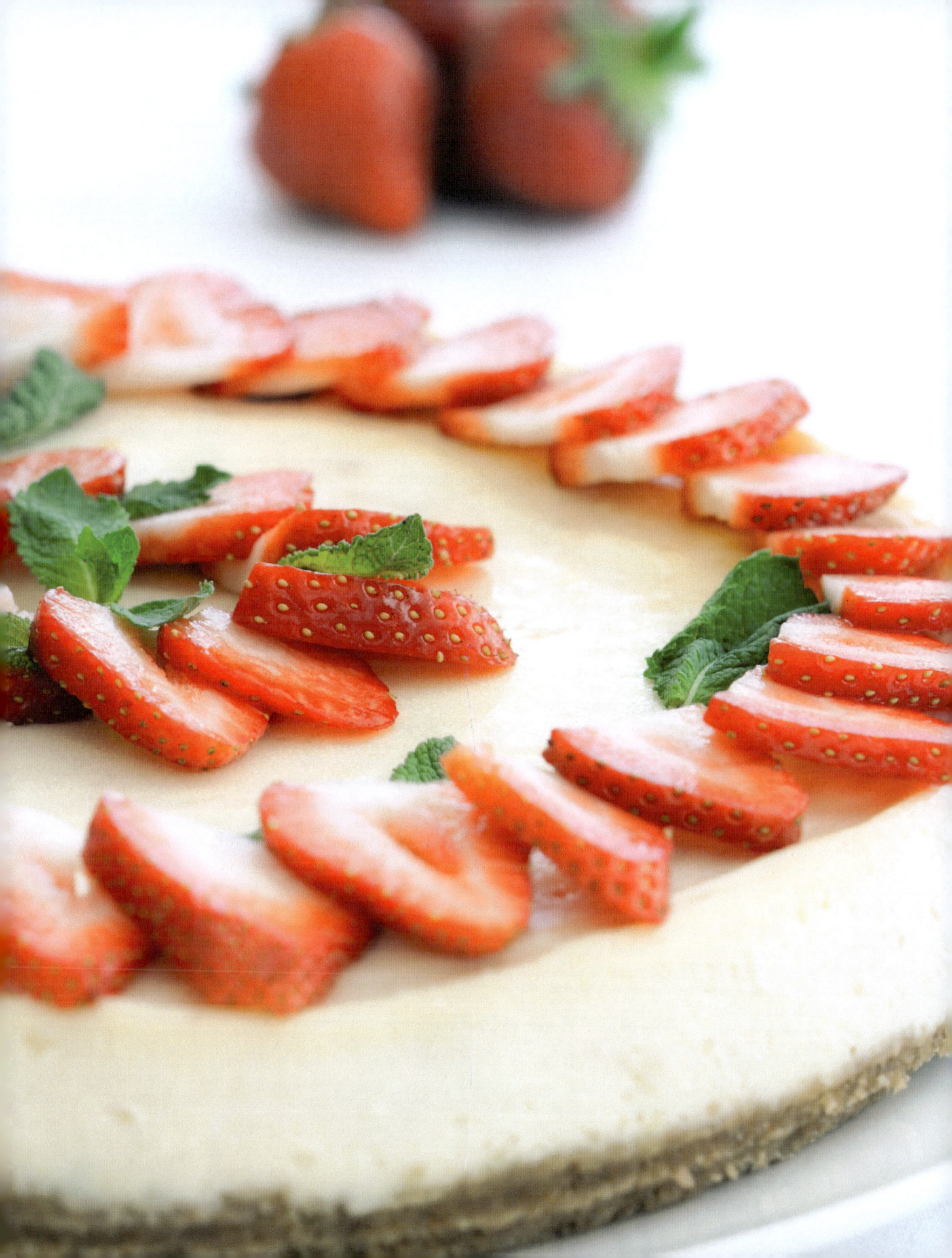

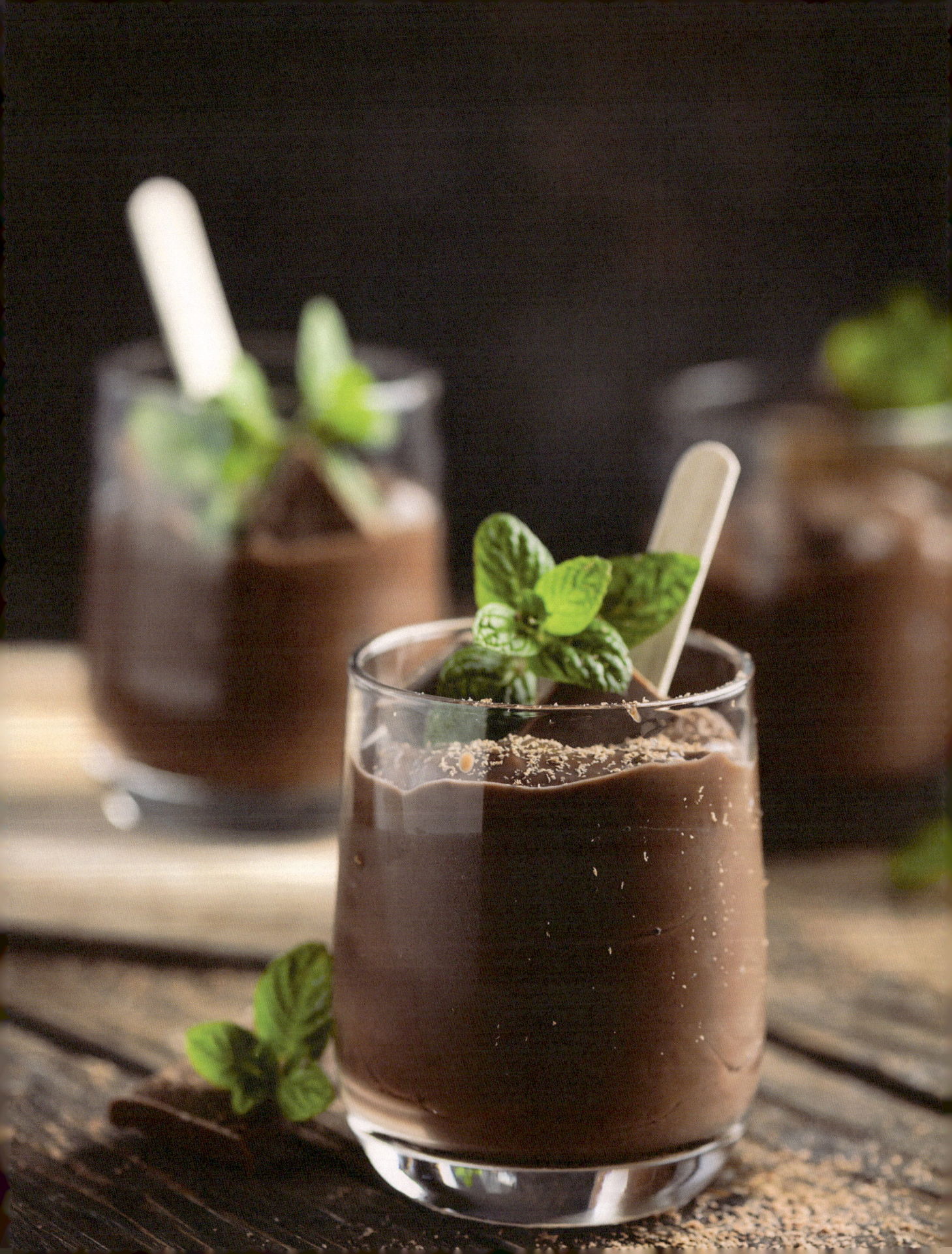

SMOOTH CHOCOLATE MOUSSE   Serves 4-6

INGREDIENTS:

5 eggs, yolk and white separated

5 tbsp caster sugar

1 1/2 tbsp butter

1 1/2 cup dark chocolate

3/4 cup double cream

Salt (to taste)

METHOD:

- Melt the butter and chocolate. Whisk the egg yolks. Heat the cream until stiff peaks form and then mix with the yolks. Fold in the melted chocolate and butter. Ensure the mix is runny but not too hot.

- Whisk the whites with the sugar until stiff peaks form. Then, fold it into the chocolate mixture until fully combined. Do not mix anymore to avoid overmixing.

- Place in a glass jars and refrigerate for at least 5 hours. Enjoy!

"Food for thought is no substitute for the real thing."

– WALT KELLY

SHORTBREAD COOKIES — Serves 6-8

INGREDIENTS:

2 cups rice flour

1 egg

1 tsp gelatin powder

1 cup caster sugar

1 tbsp vanilla extract

1 cup butter

Salt (to taste)

METHOD:

- Preheat the oven to 180°C. Bloom the gelatin by mixing it with 3 tbsp of water.
- Mix together the butter and sugar until thoroughly combined and creamy. Add in the egg, vanilla and some salt, mix, and then fold in the flour and bloomed gelatin.
- On a lined baking tray, dollop the mixture into small flattened balls, making sure to leave space between each one.
- Place in the oven for 10 minutes until slightly golden.
- When done, leave to cool and then place in the fridge for one hour before serving.

*One tip for blooming powdered gelatin, you need at least ten parts water for one part of gelatin. Using less may not allow it to bloom, using more will just thin the consistency.

SIMPLE, NO-CHURN, VANILLA ICE CREAM   Serves 4

INGREDIENTS:

2 tsp vanilla extract

2 1/2 cups double cream

1 1/3 cups condensed milk

Salt (to taste)

METHOD:

- Mix all the ingredients together by hand or with an electric whisk until the mixture becomes stiff.
- Next, transfer to a container or tin, cover and then freeze until solid (about 4-6 hours).
- Serve with ice cream or delicious on it's own.

Why not crumble in some fudge or tablet for an extra tasty treat, or serve with our fruit salad recipe?

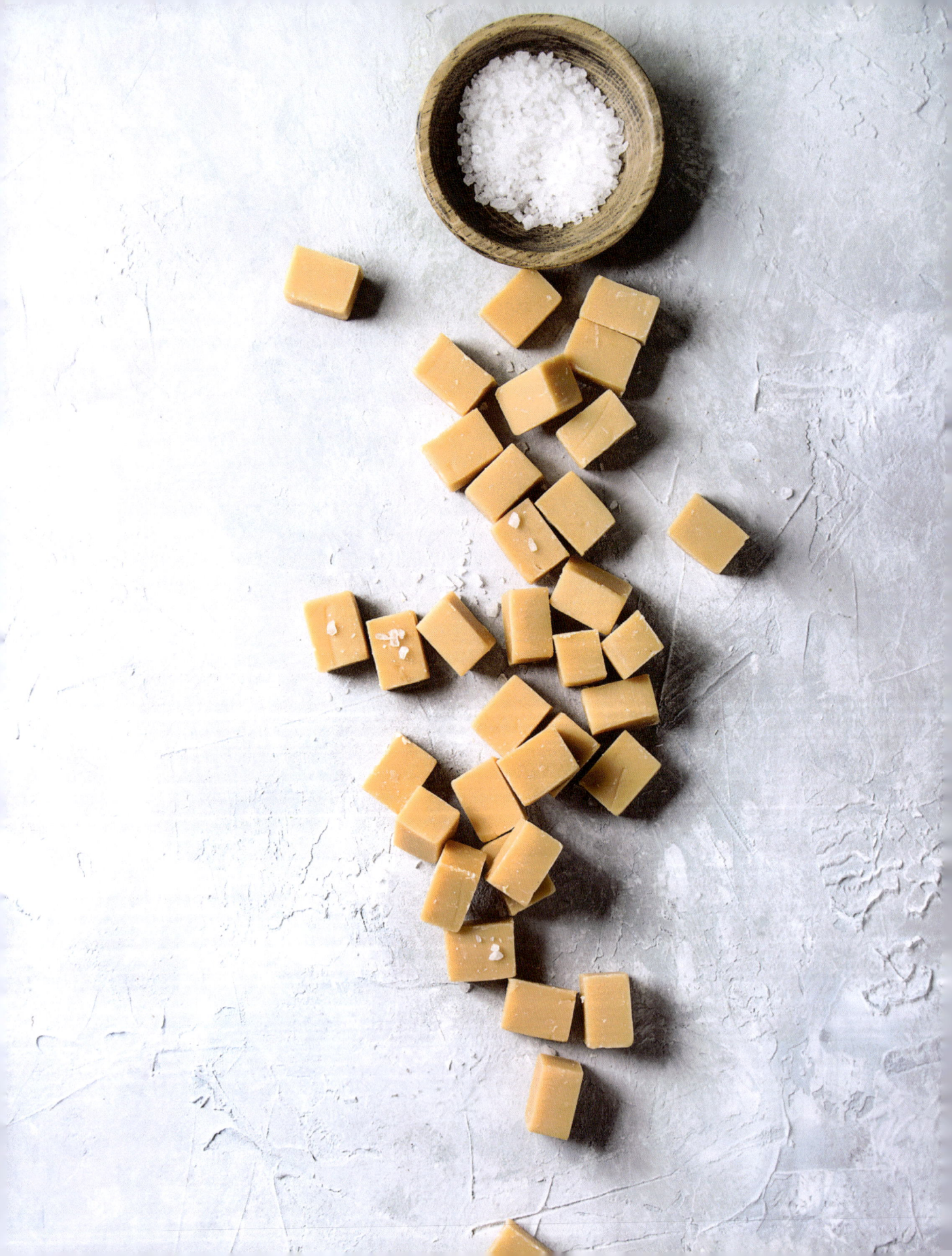

VIVACIOUS VANILLA FUDGE   Serves 6-8

INGREDIENTS:

1 1/3 cups condensed milk

1/2 cup butter

2/3 cup milk

2 tsp vanilla extract

2 1/4 cups demerara sugar

Salt (to taste)

METHOD:

- Besides the vanilla extract, place all the ingredients in a pan over a medium heat. Continuously stir as the butter melts and sugar dissolves to stop anything from burning. Keep heating until the mixture begins to boil and then slightly reduce the heat to a simmer for 10 minutes.

- To test if the fudge has reached 'soft-ball stage' and is ready, drop a small amount in a bowl of cold water. Pick it out, it should be soft, but not sticky, to touch, and you should be able to fashion it into a small 'squidgy' ball.

- If sticky, continue to simmer. If ready, remove from the heat, mix in the vanilla extract and allow the mixture to cool for 10 minutes.

- Next, beat the mixture for about 3-5 minutes until it becomes thick and loses its shine. Heating the mixture for longer will produce more crumbly fudge so use this to decide how long you want to mix it for.

- Transfer into a lined tin and flatten. Refrigerate until set (about 3 hours).

- When ready, slice into cubes and enjoy! Serve with additional salt if desired.

JOYFUL JELLY — Serves 6-8

INGREDIENTS:

3 tbsp gelatin powder

6 cups fresh fruit juice (e.g. orange)

2 tbsp honey

Salt (to taste)

METHOD:

- Mix 1 cup of juice with the gelatin powder and then allow to sit for 5 minutes so that the gelatin can bloom. The granules should swell and the mixture will look thick and lumpy.

- Meanwhile, add the rest of the juice and some salt to a pan and heat gradually until boiling. Once boiled, stir in the gelatin mix and the honey until fully dissolved.

- Transfer to a flat glass container or baking dish and refrigerate until set (around 3 hours).

- When ready, slice up and enjoy!

For an extra twist, why not add some chopped fruit pieces into the jelly mixture before it sets!

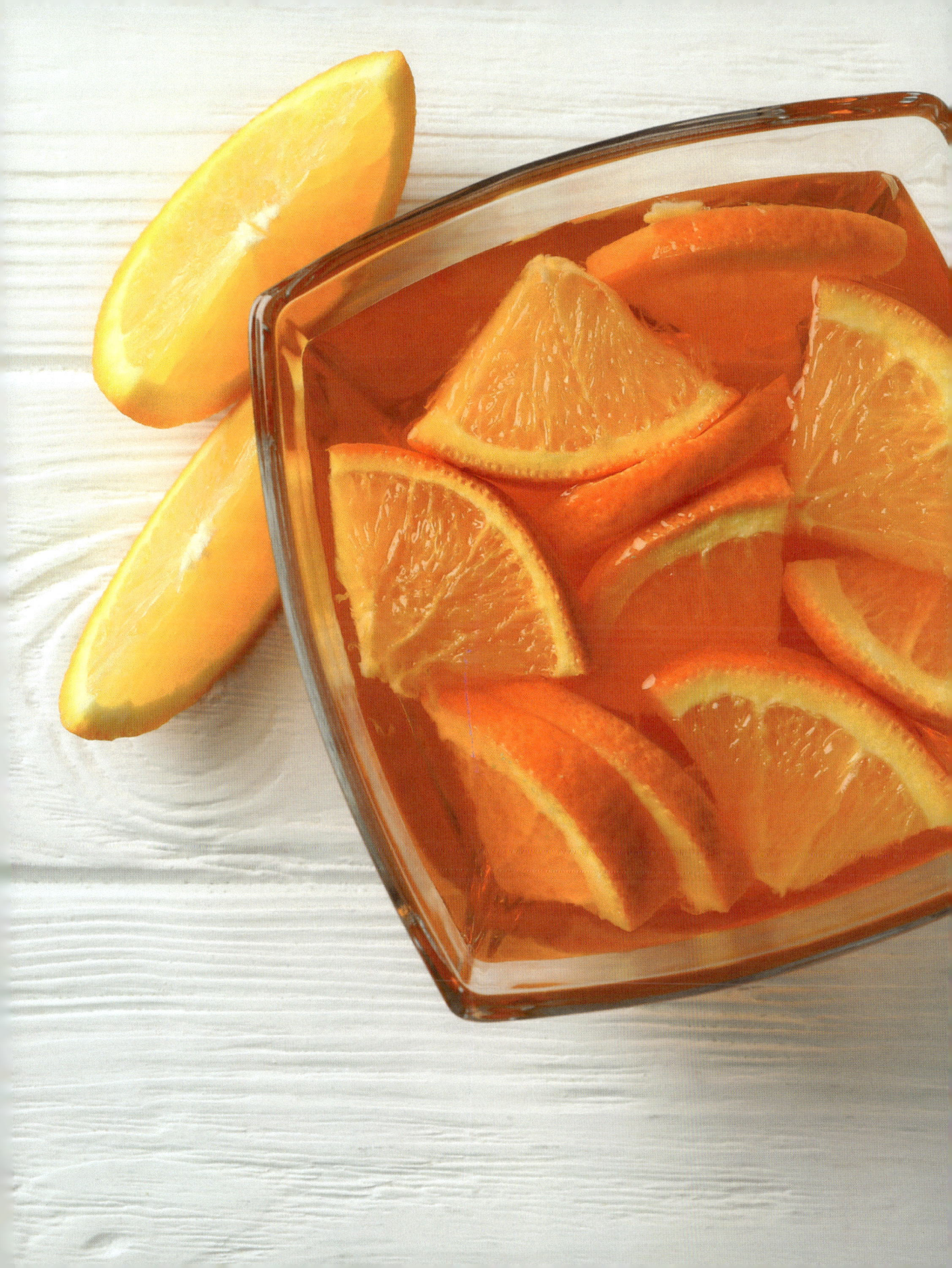

SCOTTISH CRUMBLY TABLET — Serves 6-8

INGREDIENTS:

4 1/2 cups caster sugar
1 cup milk
1/2 cup butter
1 1/3 cups condensed milk
Salt (to taste)

METHOD:

- Gently heat the milk, sugar and some salt in a pan. Regularly stir the mixture. After the sugar has dissolved, add in the butter. Once melted, add in the condensed milk.

- Continue to stir and bring the mixture to the boil. If any of the mixture starts to brown then turn down the heat. Boil until it reaches soft ball stage (see vanilla fudge recipe for details on this). The mixture should have reduced and turned golden in colour.

- Once ready, remove the pan from the heat and let it sit for 5 minutes. Then, rigorously stir the mixture until it appears to be almost setting or getting thicker. This may take about 10 minutes.

- Finally, transfer the mixture to a lined tin and flatten. Refrigerate until set (about 3 hours).

- When ready, break into pieces, savour and enjoy!

"Those who think they have no time for healthy eating. They will sooner or later have to find time for illness."

— EDWARD TANLEY

Ensure to make the time and take the time to eat like an EndoBoss®.

To your health!

Wendy xx

For further expert support
and guidance please visit

www.HealEndometriosisNaturally.com

or email

Support@HealEndometriosisNaturally.ZohoDesk.com

Printed in Great Britain
by Amazon